Where's my mum now?

Children's perspectives on helps & hindrances to their grief

Brian Cranwell

"You have made a valuable contribution to our understanding of the problems of bereaved children"
Professor Colin Murray Parkes

Illustrations by Prisca Furlong

authorHOUSE®

AuthorHouse™ UK Ltd.
500 Avebury Boulevard
Central Milton Keynes, MK9 2BE
www.authorhouse.co.uk
Phone: 08001974150

© 2010 Brian Cranwell. All rights reserved.

No part of this book may be reproduced, stored in a retrieval system, or transmitted by any means without the written permission of the author.

First published by AuthorHouse 7/19/2010

ISBN: 978-1-4490-9139-2 (sc)

This book is printed on acid-free paper.

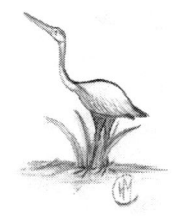

9 West View Close
Sheffield S17 3LT

Copyright
Brian Cranwell

The author wishes to thank The Child Bereavement Charity for obtaining financial support for the expenses of his enquiry, The Gone Forever Trustees for their supporting roles, Professor Emeritus Ann Faulkner for her encouragement and advice in starting and throughout this project, and the courageous children who opened their hearts to make this work possible. Finally his wife Hazel for her continuing support and encouragement.

The serial numbers in the text refer to authorities quoted in the references at the end of the book for those who wish to probe the subject more deeply. This numbering method was chosen so as to minimise interruptions in the flow of the text.

Any profits from this book after publication costs will be shared with Child Bereavement Charities

Foreword by Rt Hon David Blunkett MP

As someone who lost their father at the age of twelve in the most horrendous works accident, I can empathise with this helpful and timely publication.

For many years (including when I was Education and Employment Secretary) I worked with those campaigning to get across a greater understanding of bereavement, specifically for young people, but an understanding by adults of how this could be achieved.

In this book there is a clarity born not only of research but of empathy, which is essential for those undertaking caring professions or who have immediate and relevant contact with young people. For those in social work or as education for those positions of leadership and teaching in faith groups, this book is a timely reminder that we need to listen to children, to understand their emotional needs, and above all not to place our own anxieties and misconceptions upon them.

You will learn of the extent of bereavement for those under the age of fifteen – 18,000 losing one or more parents, in the years 2008-2009 – and understand not only the trauma and loss of bereavement, but also the lifelong scars of adults inflicting insensitive approaches for children, arising from the stress of their own ordeal.

So, in ensuring that youngsters can have their voice heard, can take part in the service, or be at the graveside, it is critical to ensure that our response and our sensitivity is informed by the experience of others. This research does just that. I commend it.

Contents

Foreword by Rt Hon David Blunkett MP	v
Introduction	1
Chapter 1. What Language?	7
Chapter 2. Anticipating a death	11
Chapter 3. Giving and receiving bad news	16
Chapter 4. To view or not to view? (The body)	23
Chapter 5. Going to the funeral and its rituals	27
Chapter 6. Back to school – the roles of teachers	37
Chapter 7. Back to school – other children's reactions	43
Chapter 8. Family influences	49
Chapter 9. Personal and Spiritual issues	60
Chapter 10. Personal change and development	66
Chapter 11. Help from outside the family	70
Chapter 12. Overprotection	76
Chapter 13. General Conclusions	81

Introduction

Much of the material in this book comes from the experiences of children interviewed for a research project at Sheffield Hallam University completed in 2007. This was the first project in the United Kingdom to seek children's own perspectives as to what has helped or hindered them prior to and following the death of a parent. 30 children ages 6 – 12 years were interviewed (17 girls and 13 boys) all of whom had known the death of at least one parent, but not including any whose deaths had been as a result of suicide, violence or a natural or other major disaster[1]. Other material comes from the author's experiences in talking to bereaved children over several years and from children's narratives in video recordings made for the London based Childhood Bereavement Network (CBN).

Although for psychological and academic reasons the research was with this particular age range and deaths of their parents, most of the principles involved apply to older and younger children, as well as to the deaths of grandparents or others close to a child, and to pets.

Helping a child through grief is not a matter of being a child psychologist or grief specialist, it is more about understanding a child's needs and the most useful ways to respond to them. Clearly the parent or immediate carer will have the most influence on this, with the school, where friendships and behaviour are important to the child and the teachers, a close second. After all, a child will spend one third of waking hours there during term time.

Every 27 minutes in this country, a father or mother of a child under the age of 15 years dies, amounting to nearly 20,000 in a year.[2] If we add those who lose a brother or sister this total comes to nearly a quarter of a million. In addition:

- Half a million have to deal with the death of a close friend.
- Over 1 million with the death of a grandparent.

UK CHILDREN'S EXPERIENCES OF DEATH

Two million children ages 5-15 years have experience of loss, many more than one.
A child loses a parent in the UK every 27 minutes = c. 20,000 a year

Grandparents (1,000,000)
Close Family/Friend (500,000)
Parent or Sibling (300,000)

As can be seen from the chart this gives a total of around two million bereaved children at any one time. Given these numbers it is not surprising (nor is it always appreciated) that:

- Some will have emotional and/or physical health problems[3]
- Many will find difficulty in concentrating
- A large number of agencies have sprung up in recent years to assist bereaved children[4]

What is appreciated even less is that there are frequently behavioural problems that arise from bereavement when adult responses are not appropriate or when no help is given.

As one child put it:

> 'Adults don't help when they don't listen to children's opinions. They make decisions for them when they don't know.' (Louise, 10)

The above figures specifically refer to the death of someone close. They do not include a parent lost through separation from a marriage or partnership, or desertion, which, depending on the circumstances and contacts, can be as traumatic, if not more so, than a death.

Health

In the past few years research has discovered that:

- Half of all children who have a parent die find difficulty in ordinary every day functioning during the first year after the death, with one in five of these needing specialist help.
- 16% of bereaved children have concentration problems one year on (compared with 6% non-bereaved).[5]
- One in five will show no signs of difficulty in the weeks immediately following a death, but confuse those around them by showing them two years later![6]

When it comes to physical health we also know that:

- Bereaved children consult G.P.'s more frequently both before and after the death of a sick parent, often for symptoms for which no medical cause can be found
- Bodily complaints in the form of an increase in infections, headaches, bed wetting, stomach upsets, sore muscles, and loss of appetite are all known to appear in some grieving children
- Some children show symptoms that are the same as those in the illness of the deceased.[7]

Compare the above with the common assumption that these problems disappear one year after the first anniversary of a death.

Effects on behaviour

Physical and emotional problems arising from grief are more generally recognised today than in the past, but less well known are the consequences of not dealing with them. For example:

- As long ago as 1966 it was found that nearly one in four children excluded from school had bereavement problems.[8] As the divorce rate has quadrupled since then it is a safe conclusion that the number of children with anger arising from adult behaviour that involves loss has increased also.

Home Office studies also show that school exclusion often sees the start of delinquent or criminal activities

- 47% losing one parent have tried drugs
- Girls losing a parent in childhood are 40% more likely to become pregnant by the age of 18 years[9]
- 20% of the children in a survey had experienced bullying at school arising directly from the death of a parent

These figures indicate a cost to the health services and to society in general. Early help for such children would require much less expense than that required, for example, for binge drinking, and result in better communication within families, with better self esteem in children.

Other Effects

As I explore in more detail in the pages that follow, in addition to the effects of bereavement on health and behaviour, it can also effect a child's academic progress, and responses and interactions with peers and families.

Assumptions

The statistics shown above in themselves would justify help to bereaved children, but there are also many assumptions about child grief by parents and others including teachers and clergy.[10] They include:

- The grief of adults does not affect the bereaved child
- Adults should avoid topics that cause a child to cry
- An active playing child is not a grieving child
- Infants and toddlers are too young to grieve
- Adults, teachers and clergy are always prepared and qualified to give instant explanations about loss, grief, and spirituality
- Children should not attend funerals.

These assumptions, (still heard quite frequently in discussions such as whether a child should attend a funeral, or be dissuaded from talking about someone who has died), together with the statistics quoted above, are the reasons for this book.

What are often referred to as the processes of grief are well researched, extensively published (in materials that can be obtained from the list at the end of this book) and are not difficult to understand, so explanations in depth are not given here.

Basically, they are much the same as for adults – shock, disbelief, anger, guilt, searching, yearning, disorganisation, despair, rebuilding and healing. Depending upon the child's age an understanding of the concept of death is also needed, and after the death opportunities for finding ways to remember the dead person so that they can move on and not be afraid to love or trust again.

The following chapters deal with these matters following the sequences of the events that occur around a death, and what can be done by those involved to assist a child before and after each event. The quotations too are drawn mainly from the children interviewed for this project. So the sequence is:

- The language we use
- Anticipating a death
- Giving and receiving bad news
- Viewing the body
- Funerals – preparing and attending
- Returning to school and other children's reactions
- Family influences
- Children's personal development and beliefs
- Help from outside the family

Chapter 1. What Language?

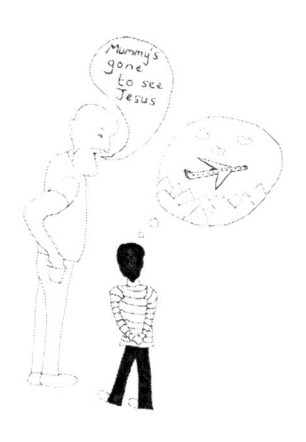

'Sometimes, it's like dad saying that everything is alright when they know that in some way it's not. It's just nice to tell the truth so it's just over with...like great grandma (Geegee, that's what I called her) when I was about five they said 'Geegee has gone, she's just gone' I didn't know what they meant, 'gone'. Gone on holiday, gone away?

It would be quite nice if they just said 'she's dead' Then, you'd like, cry but then it's over and done with and you don't have to wait another two years (sic) until they say 'Who are you looking for?' and you say 'Geegee, she went on holiday' 'Oh, sorry forgot to tell you, she died'

Whether or not they had experienced an earlier death in their families than that for which the interview took place, in almost every case these children had known a pet die. Whereas some clearly remembered their parent saying 'Jimmy's died' (the cat or the gerbil) others recalled *'they said he'd gone to sleep, but we knew what had happened anyway.'* Michael (10) added *'Gone to sleep seems kinder – but it doesn't change anything'*. Asked if he thought it was better to talk about having died more straightforwardly, he replied '

> *'I think it is. I know I do because it's like, a lot easier for me than if she says like, 'he's gone to sleep' then a couple of weeks later she says he's died and he's not going to wake up'*

The importance of using clear and logical language and of

telling the truth, when giving information and breaking bad news came across from several of the children. Although showing a tolerance of such phrases as 'Gone to sleep' Pat (10) reflected on her earlier life fears of going to bed when this had been used.

> *'When I was about six, I used to think oooooooooooo....do I have to go to sleep, can't I just stay up?'*

This preference for clear unambiguous language came across very clearly, together with an understanding of how metaphors can mystify younger children.

> *'I knew what they meant when they said 'passed away', but my young brother was a bit confused'*

Some children told of experiencing the same reactions from others, whether children or adults, as many adults experience when they or the people they are with start talking about the deceased. They assume that, even though the bereaved person brought up the subject in the first place, they will be upset so the listener tries to change the subject as quickly as possible. As Louise (9) put it:

> *My friends think, like, it is frightening for me to talk about my mum, but it's not.*

Other children were left with no confusing or ambiguous information and seemed unaware that others had such problems. This was especially true of two brothers (8 and 12) who had been brought up on a farm and had assisted with lambing or calving that included still births, or been present when a vet had humanely destroyed an animal.

Conclusions and recommendation

The use of euphemisms to hide something unpleasant is so common in English culture that we don't think about it a great deal, so consequently do not realise that children can take what we say literally. This does not only apply to the language of dying and death.

The example quoted above of the child being frightened of going to sleep is a well identified result of the use of sleep when referring to death with the resulting fear of never waking up again[11]. It is clear from the examples quoted that most children prefer straight talking.

Another reason for avoiding euphemisms is that the way we are taught to speak about death and the ways adults around us deal with the subject early in life affect the way we deal with it in later life. Teachers who tackle this sensibly find that a simple explanation as to what death means is a good starting point, especially for young children who may not realise the permanence of it. We need never assume that children cannot cope with knowing the truth.

> *Teacher: 'Sit down everyone, around me. I'm afraid I have some bad news for you this morning that we are all sad about. This is Jimmy our gerbil who has died during the weekend. As you can see he is completely still. He is not breathing and cannot see or hear, and his heart has stopped beating. He will never move again'*
>
> *Child: Can we touch him miss?*
>
> *Teacher: 'No it's best not to, we don't know what he died of, and he's all cold and stiff. We will bury him out in the garden shortly in this little box'*

Religious euphemisms are quite popular with some people, but again, these can be misinterpreted. Some statements intended to convey a sense of an after life arising from a faith can lead a child to believe the loved one elected to die. Youngsters told that 'daddy has gone to see Jesus', can lead to the conclusion that he had left the family by choice.

A favourite still in some places is the idea 'God takes the best ones first', usually an attempt at paying a compliment to the deceased as a comfort to those grieving, by saying 'It is not that he deserved to die' This not only has no justification in religious traditions, but can leave the child thinking '*If that's the case, I'll make sure I'm not next'* leaving the parent or guardian wondering why the child's behaviour has changed for the worse.

Mac (11) learned of the death of his father (separated from his mother) when an hysterical grandmother pointed to the sky while howling 'He's up there, he's up there!' conveying the idea of heaven or an afterlife being a place above the clouds.

Euphemisms are not used to confuse intentionally but are observed by those children who are old enough to be sensitive to these issues as being an adult method of talking in a kind way about death. While the older children are tolerant of them they prefer straight talk, but their use can cause confusion in younger children (seven years or under).

The conclusion we can draw from the evidence in the research programme is that failing to tell the truth in any of the matters surrounding a death, and hiding behind euphemisms or ambiguity can affect trust levels between adults and children.

Summary

Those without the experience of loss or bereavement of a parent or other significant person need:

- To receive appropriate responses through the home about loss and bereavement when a pet dies, when a friend moves away, or when any loss occurs such as moving house.
- To receive appropriate teaching at school on how everything that lives has a life span which eventually ends, how changes affect us all, and how such changes affect us emotionally and practically.[12]

Chapter 2. Anticipating a death

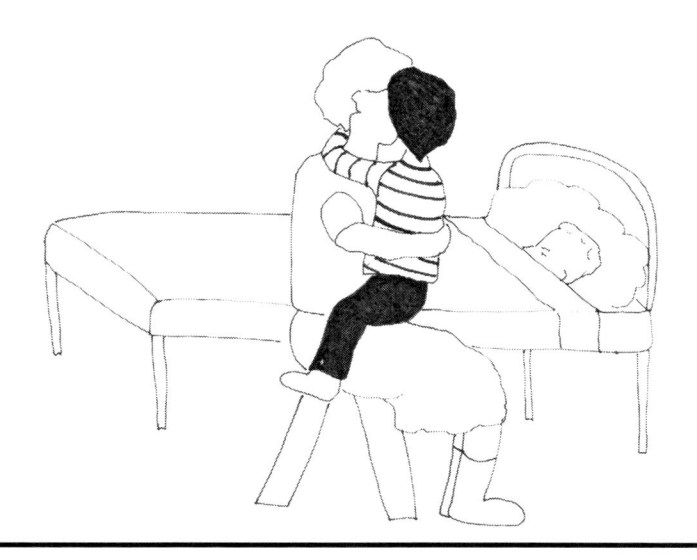

> *My mum said 'You're my beautiful girl and I'm very proud of you' then she said 'We'll meet again' because she knew she was dying (Pat, 9)*

Those who knew that their parent was dying, and knew that the parent also knew, spoke of the sense of freedom they had when talking to this parent, and to others about her. Ruth, for example, was able to discuss with her mother what life would be like without her, while Jill recalled the conversations with her mother about her dad being ill and possibly near death. Asked if she felt this had been helpful she replied

> *'It felt better to let things out, to tell the truth'*

Sometimes these conversations can take a more pragmatic and practical turn, often a feature of children's reactions. Pat recalled:

> *'I asked her if I could have a couple of animals….. and I said 'Can I still have a horse?' (giggled) and she went like, 'If you're very good!'*

Sarah knew that her father (separated from her mother and living elsewhere) was very ill and had discussed with her mother the possibility of his death so the actual event was not a complete shock. Although her brother had the same information he did not discuss this possibility with his father but was clearly pleased that he had used the opportunities of their meetings (which meant considerable travelling) to discuss his own future and plans in such a way that enabled his father to give him encouragement and affirmation.

Even finding out by accident enabled the relationship between two siblings and their terminally ill father to become more positive and constructive. They overheard him speaking on the telephone to his doctor about his prostate cancer. Their mother had died some eight years earlier.

> 'I heard him speaking to someone...I think a doctor...me and my sister was there....we found out. We started crying, so my dad just put the phone down and ran upstairs. We said 'Why didn't you tell us"?
>
> (David, 11)

Since the only other adult around was a woman friend of their fathers who seems to have been itinerant and hostile to the children, they saw themselves thereafter as his carers until he died. David observed

> 'I felt guilty at not being able to do more for him, and I think he was feeling guilty because he wasn't able to do the things that dads do'

He and his sister (14) expressed great satisfaction at the way they were given the status of carers by Health and Social Services. Whether this was an official or unofficial status does not matter.

The two brothers (10 &12) living on a farm experienced a clear case of being given false hopes whether intentionally or not. Their father had been going to hospital three times a week for some months and then sleeping when he came home, so that the family were doing all the work on the farm. Although they knew he was very ill, they had not expected him to die.

> 'Lots of people said they were making a new drug but they had only tested it on animals and they were going to get people into groups and try the drug on them, but he died before they could have that. We had hopes for this new drug.'

Another child also said her mother denied that the sick father was likely to die, again raising false hopes and increasing the shock when it happened. Only one child, Melanie, was told by her terminally ill parent of his condition.

> '... every single person in the family was in the room. And daddy was in his chair with his leg up. And I was talking to my mum and to my auntie J. and when I was talking my dad interrupted and he said I've got something to tell you, and he told me. Then grandma and granddad didn't stay in the living room, they went into the kitchen.
>
> He said 'I've got cancer and they can't get it away,' so I started crying, daddy started crying, then mummy started crying. Then mummy went out of the room and she came back in and we all had a cuddle.'

Of the children interviewed, one third of the parental deaths were very sudden (accidental, or sudden heart or respiratory attacks) and so anticipating the death and preparing them for it was not possible. Of the others, just under half were warned. Three of these spoke of the second parent or other close relative warning them of the possibility of the sick parent dying without stating outright that death was more probable than not. Pat (9), for example, whose mother had cancer, was told by her father;

> 'My dad said "some people live and some people die" and I thought, well I can't expect anything. Because you can't choose. It's a disease'

Denzil was similarly warned by his mother's sister

> 'Everyone has to die sometime'

Although not the most direct of signals, this does seem to have given some preparation. Alan too felt he had been warned by inference by his grandmother though he could not remember the exact words. The rest were either told nothing or given false hopes.

Conclusions and recommendations

Knowing in advance that someone close is dying created two conditions observable in this survey. Firstly it enabled some of the children involved to have discussions with the dying parent that they will probably remember and treasure all their lives, an example of which (Pat) was given above. Secondly the sense of freedom that this knowledge invoked was clear in talking to them even two years after the events. Even the brother and sister who found out by accident were pleased they had done so.

However, these same two children brought up a point with their father at the time of discovery that is a significant lesson. The question '*Why didn't you tell us?*' reflected not only anger, but in the interview conversation the question of trust was raised.

As with the avoidance of euphemisms, the reactions of those children warned of impending death does indicate that children can cope with the truth if they grow up with it. It clearly gave the children who were warned and prepared a sense of being treated in a grown up way and being trusted. Being told the truth enables the children to be given and feel support through the period when grief is anticipated, thus enabling them to begin working through their pain. Without such preparation all the bad news – sickness, death, moving to mortuary, funeral parlour, funeral, empty place at the table and adjustment to living permanently without the deceased– is heaped on the child within a few days.[13]

Being told the truth also ensures that the child feels it is being treated as an equal member of the family. Anybody who has worked with bereaved children will have come across situations, where a child receives sympathy from a neighbour or someone else outside of the family and hears such words as 'Of course, we knew your dad was very ill and hadn't got long to go'. This can leave the child thinking 'How is it they knew and I wasn't told?'

A Head Teacher made a comment that reflected several on the same issue heard from a number of adults over the years, showing how memories of these events when not handled sensitively can be retained as negative experiences possibly for the rest of life.

> *'I adored my gran and still remember the fact that nobody told me she was ill and was going to die. Forty years on I still find myself thinking about her and the fact that I never had a chance to say goodbye'*

Summary

For children with a parent who is terminally ill:

- To be told the truth, especially when it is evident that the sick person is coming to the end of their life. To be given the chance to talk to the dying and the surviving parent and discuss the issues involved for them all.
- If the dying parent is the only parent, for that parent or others in the family to ensure that all possible legal procedures are in place to ensure that the wishes of the dying parent with regard to the future care of the child are carried out with the consent of those involved and the child.

Chapter 3. Giving and receiving bad news

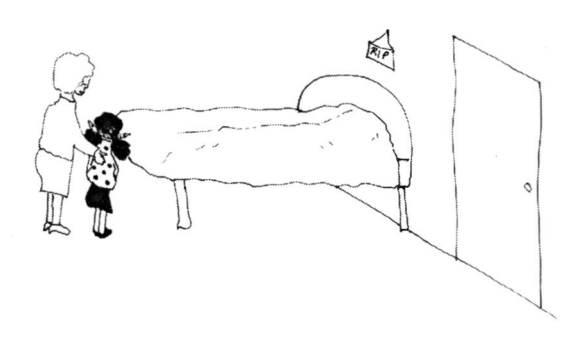

> '*When mum put me into this car she didn't say owt. She laughed and said "It's just a fancy car, it's taking us somewhere", and I just ended up at the funeral. Then she went "oh it's your dad, and I went "ooooooooh" just like that. When I got to the cemetery I thought we was going to see me nanan, and she said, " No, your dad's died" so that's how I found out about it'.* (Jill,7)

Two thirds of the children interviewed were told of the death by the surviving parent, though in the case quoted above the circumstances can only be described as bizarre. Jill's father had been in hospital several weeks and she and the other siblings had been with their mother to see him 3 – 4 times a week. There came a day when their mother said he was too ill to talk to them so they did not go again. The following Friday they did not go to school as their mother said they were going out. A black limousine arrived during the morning, and the events described above followed. Jill reported that she was so upset that she had to be carried into the church, but then, remarkably, at some point during the service she went forward and stood by the coffin and said a prayer of thanksgiving for all her daddy had done and meant to her.

The children interviewed could be grouped as follows:

Nearly one third were with the parent at a time of very sudden death with no warning. Of these nearly half were alone with the deceased at the time but not one was subsequently advised of the cause of death, and only half the others knew the actual cause. The other half knew the cause since the emergency nature at the time of death was related to a lingering condition that the parent had suffered with for some time, such as asthma. Among these were children who were not told by the surviving parent, or were told by someone else because they had become orphans.

None of the others told directly by their surviving parent were told in the dramatic fashion described in the opening box. Two or three told of having the news broken the following morning since their parent felt it unhelpful to wake them up in the night for this purpose, and they were content with this. One (Pat) learned by overhearing her relatives in a state during the evening after going to bed, following a 'phone call from her mother's hospital.

11 year old Dick's father displayed a sensitive approach after his mother had been taken to hospital the previous night with a heart attack.

> 'My dad brought me and my brother into his bedroom, and he said um, last night as you know your mum was feeling really ill and unfortunately she had a really bad asthma attack, and she passed away, that was when it really hit me, she'd gone'

Most parents gave the news in a direct and sensitive way as far as these children remembered along the lines

> 'I'm afraid I've got some bad news for you. Your mum has died'

Of the one third not told by the surviving parent, one was told by the police (in the presence of his mother). This one, and some of those telling their stories in a CBN video, were affirming of the way the police handled this task, speaking of officers *'telling how it is and speaking directly'*

Those told by other relatives did not all have very good experiences. Mac, (11) mentioned earlier as being told by his hysterical grandmother, had been taken to see her by his mother (separated from his father) who already knew of his father's death. Hazel (9), whose mother had been in hospital some weeks was woken up by her elder brother, who had been to the hospital to see their mother the previous evening with their father.

> *'My dad didn't tell me the same night. I woke up and then my brother kept on saying it (that their mother had died) but I didn't believe it, and I said "Stop lying, 'cos it's serious".*
>
> *And then my dad was on his mobile talking to somebody and I shouted him that and he said it was real, and then I was really shocked and started crying'*

Abigail's (10) experience when told by her older sister of the death of their mother, bordered on the humorous for adult ears. She and her younger brother had been fostered for some months as when her mother took ill their father had walked out. The mother had spent some months in hospital where she was when Abigail went on holiday with her fostering couple. She returned to find her sister waiting for them.

> *She said 'I've got some bad news and some good news. The bad news is that mum has died. The good news is she left us £300 that we can either spend or use it for her gravestone'*

Abigail did not find any difficulty with this announcement, and they agreed to use the money for a gravestone.

Conclusions and recommendations

The fact that many of the children whose parent died suddenly while they were present did not know the cause of death is itself a cause for concern. Children these days watch television programmes such as 'Casualty'; and see people restored to life by having pressure applied to their chest, and feel they should have been able to do something to help. Where the death has come about through violence children who are present also frequently believe they should have done something to prevent it.

Small children often experience what is called 'magical thinking' whereby they believe they have brought about the death of someone close either by malevolent thoughts ('I hate you!') or because they had been naughty or disruptive.[14]

It is therefore very helpful for a child to be reassured that everything possible was done for the dead parent, by nearest and dearest, by the ambulance staff, the doctors and nurses, and that there was nothing the child could have done to help the deceased.

There were indicators that some adults would have preferred to say nothing to the children. As with most mistaken assumptions such actions, or lack of them, are seldom if ever taken other than the adult concerned believing they are protecting the child. But lack of information can not only be worrying for a child, it can be injurious.

Terry had just started school as a five year old. One evening his mother put him to bed at his usual time, in the room he shared with his 18 months old younger brother.

After a while Terry got out of bed, lifted his brother out of his cot and played with him. Their mother heard them, came in, scolded Terry severely and put them both back into their beds.

The next day Terry came back from school to find that every

trace of his young brother had disappeared and he was not allowed to ask questions or talk about him. This left him convinced that he had caused the child to go away or die. It was not until 30 years later when his mother died and he helped his father clear out her personal belongings that he found newspaper cuttings indicating that the baby had died a cot death.

His wife told the author that Terry had never let a day go by without mentioning his little brother, and had suffered from depression most of his adult life. He committed suicide leaving a family of four children aged 5 – 14 years.

Bad news is still bad news however sensitively the information is given, but it is clear that the children appreciated straight talking. Giving the news in a comfortable place away from a hospital ward is preferable to being in the ward or in the corridor outside. The process of starting with such words as *'I'm afraid I have some bad news for you'* is at least a warning that something unpleasant is coming. Wherever possible it is best delivered by someone close to or trusted by a child, in a private situation without haste, and where there are no barriers that will prevent contact if the child needs to cry and be cuddled. Tissues on hand will also be useful.[15]

The lack of knowledge by Social Workers, not only of resources that would be helpful to the foster parent of a grieving child, but where to find such help, and the reactions of two Social Work Managers to these interviews, one on the grounds that the child had been consulted by a school mentor who knew the family well, before the Social Worker (who hardly knew him at all) indicates a lack of training in this field that seems inappropriate for people with responsibilities for bereaved children's placements and welfare. In addition, siblings I interviewed who went straight into care after their second parent died were not consulted about the disposal of their family's personal effects. The result was that a girl friend of their father's who was living with them, and who was very hostile to the children, disposed of everything herself and the children do not have so much as a photograph of either parent.

Finally, when parents are separated, it is important for the surviving parent to remember that whatever happened between the parents is not the fault of the child, to express regret at their loss and assure them that the deceased parent still loved them. There were no instances of outright hostility being expressed about the dead parent in this study (although the mother who left it to her mother-in-law to tell Mac seems to have stood back from the responsibility) but most people who work with bereaved children have heard of situations where a child has been caused further upset by bitter words by the surviving parent or others.

One child has no idea where her father is buried or his ashes are placed because her grandparents were so bitter about their son's marriage break up that they refused to tell his family where or when the funeral was to be held and the whereabouts of his remains. This is a clear case of vindictiveness against an innocent party. There is nothing this child wanted more in life than to be able to go to her father's grave.

As leading psychiatrists[16] have pointed out, children of separated parents frequently have secret hopes that their parents will reunite as a family. When one dies they have a double loss, the loss of the parent and the loss of this hope.

Summary

For children who have a parent die, with one surviving:

- To receive the information about the death in an appropriate manner directly from the surviving parent (where possible).
- If the surviving parent is unable to break the news (through separation or illness) to decide in advance of the death who is to advise the child it has happened.
- To assure the child that everything possible was done

for the deceased and that the child was in no way responsible.
- To reassure the child that the state of relationships between the parents did not alter the fact of the deceased being the child's parent and their love for the child.

When the child has no surviving parent:

- If the child is to be in the care of Social Services and Foster Parents, having social workers and carers who understand the needs of bereaved children.
- That foster parents are provided with appropriate information.
- and literature that will enable them to understand something of the child's problems, and where to go for help.
- To ensure that whoever is responsible for disposal of the belongings of the last parent ensures that the child is included in the distribution or disposal of photographs, and personal items that will enable a continuing memory and bond with the deceased.

Chapter 4.. To view or not to view? (The body)

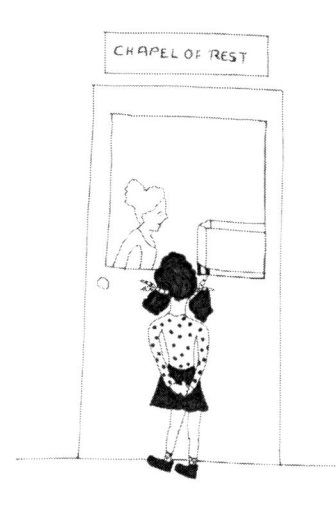

> 'I was pleased I went in. All the pain had gone from her face'

Abigail, (10) whose mother had been in hospital several months and had suffered with cancer for two years made her own decision to go to see her mother's body when her aunt gave her the option. As she indicated above and later expressed clearly, had she not done so her abiding memory would have been of someone continually in pain.

Ricky too remembered how pleased he was to have seen his mum;

> 'It made me feel better just seeing her again. It felt just right to be honest, just seeing her and saying goodbye'

Julia, whose parents and sibling were killed in a road accident abroad, from which she was the sole survivor, could not view the damaged bodies, so they were placed in sealed coffins in the kitchen of their home the night before the funeral. Julia spent an hour with them accompanied by her parish priest and she shared her memories with him and said prayers;

> 'I felt really close to them and that we had said goodbye to each other'

Louise did express a wish to see her mother's body but was refused. She came across as quite angry about this:

> 'Adults don't help when they don't listen to children's opinions. They make decisions for them when they don't know'

One third of the children in the survey were given the option of viewing their parent's body. Of these twice as many chose to do so as chose not to, while a similar number would have liked to view but were not given the option.

The children who were with the parent at time of death or who died suddenly at home can be added to those who saw their bodies, but none of these saw them again before the funeral.

Melanie (8), arrived at the hospice where her father had been a patient ten minutes after he died and heard talk of his death. She was determined to satisfy herself, so accompanied by her grandmother went to his bed and felt his pulse.

> 'I started crying when I tried to do his pulse and then one of my tears dropped on him'

Having satisfied herself he was dead she then pulled the blankets up to cover him up to his shoulders.

> 'And then I ……. kissed him and his lips were very black'

When she first saw him she thought he was sleeping. Asked if she would have been less upset if she had been told instead of seeing him she replied:

> 'I'd be much upset if they told me because I would have found out for myself anyway'

One grandmother, looking after her four year old grand daughter, related how the child insisted on going to see her father's body when told of his death. Reluctantly she arranged this but could not take the child herself. On her return the little girl said

> *'I saw daddy. He's dead but he still had his skin on!'*

The grandmother concluded that at some stage someone had tried to explain to the child what happens after we die and she had half expected just to see a heap of bones.

None of the children who were with their parent at the time of death seemed to feel that they had experienced any particularly traumatic event, other than the usual sense of shock. Two children saw their father in intensive care on life support following a severe stroke but from the mother's comments it seemed that he was only being kept alive to allow the children to see him before switching off these machines.

Three children who did not view the body seemed to gain satisfaction from the fact that they knew that poems they had written out and favourite soft toys had been placed in the coffin.

Conclusions and recommendations

Certain parts of the United Kingdom still have traditions that involve all in a community viewing or seeing the body of a family member, as would have happened everywhere before the days of a funeral director whisking the body away out of sight to a mortuary or funeral parlour.

The evidence points to most children benefiting long term in their grief from seeing the body[17]. In some cases they need to convince themselves that the person is dead. Plus, in these days when many families split up and the children have friends at school who live with only one parent they may well have heard of other children being told a parent had died when in fact they had left home.

A survey of 318 children aged 5 – 17 years bereaved of a

parent in the USA found that 9 out of 10 viewed the body of their parent at the funeral parlour, and that this is something of a family ritual. Many of them expressed their appreciation of the music and flowers, and being able to place poems, pictures, or letters in the coffin.

Again, the natural instinct of the parent to protect their child, means that refusal is a common response, and some parents are adamant about this. Such refusal often reflects the problem of the adult over death. While it would be unwise to insist that a child sees the body (and the Funeral Director will advise if the body is fit to be seen) giving the decision to the child helps them to feel that they have an option and are believed to be mature enough to make the decision themselves.

The way the opportunity is offered can also make a difference. The invitation 'Come and hold my hand while we go to see your mum/dad, and I'll hold yours' conveys the message that the adult feels as vulnerable as the child and enables the child to feel s/he is helping the adult.

Summary

Children can be encouraged without fear of hurt, and without coercion, to see the body of the deceased. Much will depend on the fears of the accompanying adult.

The funeral director will always be ready to advise if it is not advisable to view the body in the event of visible damage

Chapter 5. Going to the funeral and its rituals

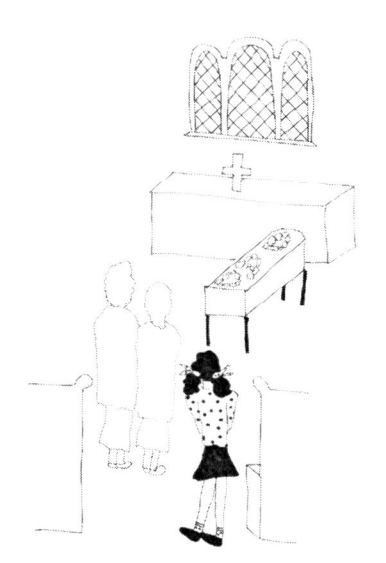

> 'I thought like, it was for my dad, and for me to go to the funeral rather than not go…. because then like, a couple of years later I probably think, why I did not go to the funeral?' Marilyn

Nearly all the children in the survey attended, an unusually high proportion compared with the experiences of most ministers questioned who typically see children at less than half of the funerals at which the presence of children could have been expected given their relationship with the deceased. In a survey done for this work the twelve ministers involved reported that only one third of the families who had children who were close to the deceased allowed these children to attend the funeral.

Marilyn, quoted earlier, had a clear idea that by not going she might store up regrets for the future. Others, such as Michael (10), who had been reluctant to go were pleased they had attended for the same reason. As Ruth (11) put it

> 'It was a nice way of saying 'Goodbye' and saying 'See you soon I guess'….. ….(laughing) 'well not too soon, but eventually'

Only one (Mabel, 12) expressed regret at having attended, not because of the funeral but because of the attitudes of some adults present who came up to her and said such things as '*Oh you poor thing*' which made her feel uncomfortable and patronised.

Jill, the 7 year old child mentioned earlier who did not know her father was dead until she arrived at the church for the funeral with her mother, was severely shocked on first hearing this but carried on into the church while weeping heavily. At some time during the service she got to her feet at the invitation of the priest, and went forward to the coffin.

> '*I got to get up and went on to the big thing (the lectern) and say (sic) something to my dad like 'I love you' and I want my mum to be OK and....and then I did a prayer by the stairs for me dad.*'

One of the most memorable features for many children was the numbers present. As all the children in the survey were 12 years or under this meant that most of the parents who had died were relatively young. As 12 year old Ricky put it

> '*What I really want you to know is that I was really quite proud because the whole church was jam packed with people, people that we knew*'

Ruth too told of her surprise at how many people were present and knew her mother.

> '*I felt- Wow, my mum is really popular*'

Leo also '*I didn't know she was that popular!* a sentiment echoed by Denzil who added '*There were people there I didn't even know!* while Sandra was even more expressive on the subject.

> '*There were so many people that I didn't even know. My teacher came whom I used to talk to. I was quite surprised about that but she came. Some of my friends came, my closest friends. My*

> *dancing teacher came, because I'm really close to her as well'*

Only one child recalled anything said at the funeral by the conductor that seemed aimed at helping the children present, and this was by the person leading the secular event for Pat's mother.

> *'these things that he said were good for children about my age, and Sarah (friend) started laughing a bit, and some others, and it was quite funny...... and he said nice things'*

Although several children felt they had contributed in some way by placing gifts, letters or cards in the coffins, less than a third had any idea as to what they expected to happen at the funeral, nor were they invited to participate. One exception was Sophie, who 'made a speech'. She could not remember what she said but remembered finishing with a poem which had a line about her mum 'being an angel without wings.'

One who did know what to expect was Pat, whose mother's funeral was a secular event.

> *'We said what music we was going to have, and we had the Labour Party music...and other things'*

Not knowing what to expect caused several children to fantasise, and have fears such as the coffin being open (as in American films). Hazel said she was surprised that the coffin was there at all while Jenni confessed to being nervous about not knowing though she was not sure why.

Among those who did know what to expect were Keith and his sister who had been briefed by their mother beforehand and who both participated. Melanie too expressed pleasure at having the opportunity to read a poem that she had written herself.

There were several expressions of appreciation at the presence of work colleagues, while Jennie remembers her father's police uniform being placed on top of the coffin. Two children expressed great appreciation that other children from their school were present accompanied by their class teacher and parents, others at the attendance of more remote family members and neighbours.

The brother and sister who were not allowed to attend their father's funeral but had to go to school, were clearly resentful (and this may have led to the boy's subsequent exclusion from school). Several authorities have found that such decisions are frequently based not on the child's needs, but on parents' own discomfort with having the children present.

Other Memories

A few of the children could remember one or two things mentioned at the funeral, especially if they caused laughter, or were stories about the deceased parent. Pat particularly remembered the person conducting the secular funeral making amusing comments, while Jenni recalled how they all laughed at the priest relating the story of how her parents became engaged.

A surprising number of verbal messages were recalled. Ruth remembers the priest saying that death comes to all of us; Hazel her dad giving an appreciation of how her mum was always there when he came home even if she only told him off; Alan remembers hearing his name, his gran's and his sister's in the address or the prayers.

Conclusions and recommendations

Many ministers consulted in this project spoke of concern at the number of children who are excluded from family funerals. The larger than usual percentage in this survey who did attend may have been because parents or guardians who were willing to allow their children to be interviewed would also be people who would be more open to their attendance, or because this survey was targeted solely at children who had lost a parent.

Figures for this will differ in different parts of the United

Kingdom where distinctive communities retain certain traditions. In parts of Wales for example there are still villages where the tradition is that men alone attend.

There is a strong assumption shown in this survey that children either know what to expect will happen, or do not need to know, even though it was clear from the children's responses that few of them, had such knowledge and in some cases were quite anxious. This is not to say that children will always remember what they are told to expect, just as adults do not remember such details in times of high tension or trauma, but the act of telling them enables them to feel trusted and an equal part of the family[18], and helps give them the belief that they will be able to cope.

The information issue is reflected again in removing pressure on a child when given the option to attend. Pat told how she had been given a book at school that included a passage that said 'if you do decide not go to the funeral you don't need to feel guilty, sometimes people don't want to go.' She found this very helpful but decided she would go, possibly as the pressure was removed. After, she felt it important that she had attended

> *'because you see what happens there instead of going around asking questions....some people think they don't know what is inside the coffin.'*

She remembers thinking

> *'My mum's in there, there's a dead body in that with my picture and the things I gave her.'*

It is clear that funerals meet similar needs in children as those in adults[19]. By being included in the rituals they felt acknowledged and supported, knew what to expect, and had an opportunity to say goodbye. Even those who had been ambivalent about attending in this sample recognised afterwards that missing the event was something they might have regretted later in life.

Only one child, David, found that he could not cope with his emotions and left the funeral service before the end, but was still pleased that he had made the effort. The rest were clearly in control, taking in various new sights and experiences but acknowledging that they were in tears and sad. Pat spoke of being in control until she found how many adults around her were in tears and these triggered off her own.

Children who experienced the presence of other children at their parent's funeral, whether from school, family members or friends and neighbours were very appreciative of this sense of being supported. Similarly, the quotes of appreciation at the attendance of so many people including friends or work colleagues also show that they recognised the value of the funeral in honouring the deceased parent, not only within the family but also in their role in society or workplace.

The survey having been carried out among children of 6 – 12 years meant that the deceased parent was usually in the 25 – 40 age group, which meant that their friends from school, college and work would be around if they still lived in the same area in which they grew up or attended college. Several children expressed their sense of pride in the numbers present, something they will retain all their lives.

One family (not included in the original study) took advantage of the trend towards eco friendly woodland burial sites by turning the funeral of the father into a family outing and picnic. Their father's body was in a cardboard coffin, and the mother provided felt tip pens. The adults wrote messages on the coffin and the children, most of whom were under 12 years, drew pictures. The coffin was lowered into the grave and the grave filled in by family members, who then all had a picnic by the grave. It was reported by one adult with a lot of funeral experiences as 'the most moving funeral ever attended.'

Summary

Children can be helped in their decision about attendance by

- Feeling that they made the decision themselves, by stressing the opportunity to make their farewells, and to see a demonstration of the popularity of the deceased by the presence of neighbours, friends and work colleagues as well as relatives.
- Explaining what will happen. (If adults are not sure themselves the minister or person conducting the funeral will usually be happy to explain)
- Being included in the planning of the funeral rites and any subsequent gathering, with the option of participating or making some contribution if desired.
- Arranging for them to sit with another relative or friend if the surviving parent or guardian feels they cannot cope with a child and their own grief.
- Taking a child to the funeral of someone they do not have a great deal of emotional involvement with. This enables them to see what happens and to have some idea as to what to expect. This is especially helpful when the likelihood of the funeral of someone close is imminent. As the handbook of Winston's Wish (one of the top advisory groups on the subject anywhere in the world) points out, children are more scared about what they don't know than what they are allowed to participate in, as this helps them feel more included.

After the funeral – the Wake

You have to have a party after a funeral and go to a pub, don't you? You have to have a party

Most of the children interviewed took it for granted that there would be some sort of gathering after the funeral and attended whether in a pub or at someone's house. All viewed this as an important and good experience and several used the word 'celebration' to describe the gathering. One or two expressed surprise at how quickly the mood changed from tears and sadness to smiles, and laughter at the wake, but did not find this upsetting as their own experience was very similar.

> 'even though they were still a little bit red around the eyes' (Pat)

They were not dismayed by this and joined in as best they could

> 'my dad said – just be happy, your mum wants you to be happy'

Those with friends or relatives of their own age group present spoke of spending most of the time playing with or talking to them

> 'Me and my friends we just went upstairs and my dad ordered some pizzas....and he said "surprise, .pizzas!"'

Those who went to a small family gathering back home where they were the only one or one of two children present, reported feeling a bit out of things as the adults tended to talk only to each other.

The only discordant note was when Jill's mother had a dispute with a relative.

> 'What made me upset was me mum and me uncle (dad's brother) weren't friends any more, and they aren't friends now'

Conclusion and Recommendations

The general view that 'Mum/dad would have wanted people to enjoy themselves' came across very strongly. It was clearly important to the children that they had participated in what they saw was a part of the ceremonies and rituals involving saying their 'goodbyes' to the deceased. The only dissident from this view was a girl whose attitude reflected that of her mother:

> *'We didn't have any sort of party after my dad's funeral. My mum thinks it's wrong to do this after the funeral of someone you love and she doesn't understand how other people can do it, and I agree with her.' (Jennie)*

The Importance of Rituals

Many of those who conduct funerals find that a lot of parents have already made up their minds that their children will not attend a funeral under any circumstances and will not be budged, believing that this will be too upsetting for a child. The suggestion that the child might be more upset by being excluded is frequently just not believed despite quoting the experiences of many adults who have felt guilty and resentful for the rest of their lives at this exclusion.

There is now ample evidence to show that the rituals of funeral attendance, viewing the body, and some sort of wake gathering provide important steps in helping the grieving process for both children and adults. One study of 120 children showed that 95% of them believed that their attendance had helped them accept the reality of their loss and receive help and comfort, regardless of whether the funeral itself had been of a religious or secular nature, whereas other studies show that children who are not given preparation and support and do not attend show more behaviour problems.[20]

Western society in many instances is abandoning the rituals and rites of passage that still exist in other cultures that help a child confirm its identity and affirm movement from childhood to adult. Being included helps a child feel acknowledged and supported and to feel accepted as an equal member of the family. The evidence also shows that a funeral helps a child acknowledge the reality of the death of someone close, enables them to honour the life of the person who has died, while supplying support and comfort provided they are briefed as to what to expect.

Those who work with bereaved children have frequently come across youngsters who are at first annoyed at not being allowed to attend, then furious when they discover that relatives they have never or hardly ever met, who have not seen their deceased parent for years and who live a long way away, turn up and are welcomed, while the child has to go to school.

Chapter 6. Back to school – the roles of teachers

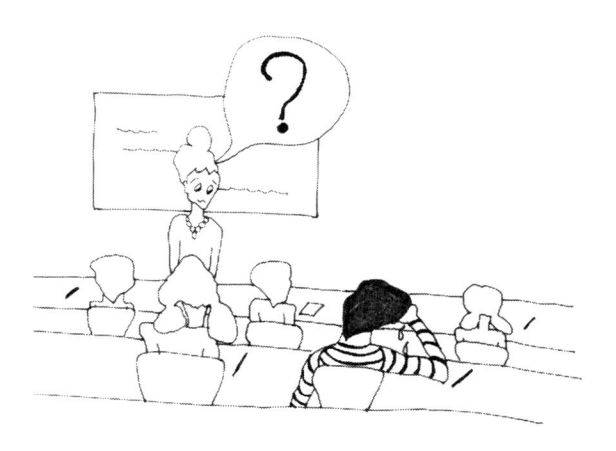

Most of the children interviewed wanted to get back to school as soon as possible after hearing of the death of their parent. Partly, they said, this was because they wanted to be with their friends and partly because they just liked to be there. But experiences varied.

> *'School, it really helped me….Miss Hake, she gets me doing lots of jobs. I'm a reading tutor for other children'*
> (David)
>
> I got bullied, like, two years in a row. The teachers didn't do anything about it……..people kept saying nasty things like "Ho ho, you haven't got a dad" (Sarah)

50% of those interviewed felt that they had received useful support from school staff, both teachers and mentors. The rest were divided equally between those who found teachers distinctly negative with little acknowledgement of their loss, and those who expressed some sympathy at first but made no effort to see if the child had any special problems with such issues as concentration, or negative responses from other children.

Mac for example was angry with his class teacher and the head following his father's death.

> *'They gave me a lot of attention at first but three weeks later another boy in my class had the same experience and the staff seemed to lose interest in me'*

In addition he recounted some unpleasant comments made to him about his father in the coach during a school trip, which he felt the staff ignored.

> *'I don't really feel like going back. They kept picking on me'*

Among the teachers expressing some initial sympathy but then moving on, their feelings were perceived by the children not so much as the staff being uncaring but conveying the impression that this was not an important or significant event in the life of the school or the class.

Some of the positive staff responses included:

- Talking to the rest of the child's class without the child present to tell them this was a sad time for him/her, to not treat him too differently from normal but be aware that there may be times when she/he will want to be alone or leave the room.
- Giving permission to leave the class for a short break when feelings overwhelm the child. *'When it happens, I don't want anyone else around me'*
- Having a system of visual signals, such as a card or stone with red on one side and green on the other displayed on the desk so that if the child turns it to

red and leaves he/she can do so without explanations (The teachers who had practised this advised that they had never known it to be abused by a child).

- Staff trained in bereavement work.

'It's got better since I've had bereavement counselling. We've got like a book, we write down a diary and everything. And then we've got these sheets. It's like a key and we colour – if you're happy it's yellow, like, how you're feeling' (Ronnie)

Jill and Kevin had bereavement counselling from the same teacher as Ronnie. *'She's just helped a lot'*

Not all experiences were as positive. Jimmy said he would have liked to go out at times but did not like to ask. Hazel said she had been told by her teacher to feel free to go out for such a break if necessary.

'but I don't think she really meant it, she wouldn't like it if I did'.

One other point made by several children, that comes across also in one of The Child Bereavement Network diary videos, is that bereaved children do not like to be made to appear 'different'. One teenager tells of how his teacher told the class that they were going to make cards for Father's Day *'But not you, Jimmy, you haven't got one. Help somebody else'* The boy went home and made one, which he then stuck on to his father's headstone.

Conclusions and recommendations

The bigger the school, the greater the probability of a death by another child or a member of staff or other losses, and various people listed at the end of the book have made suggestions for school policies, staff training, and contingency planning for such losses. It was significant that in two of the schools where the subject was discussed most freely, the two mentors who had given counselling to four of the children interviewed had attended bereavement training programmes.

It is a poor reflection on teacher training that a survey carried out for a children's hospice, which involved interviewing 250 children, showed that nearly 60% of the teachers also interviewed said they felt inadequate in dealing with bereaved children, yet nearly 80% of these schools had at least one child bereaved within the previous two years. Few of the schools involved had any bereavement policies in place.[21]

Because school is often seen by a child as a safe, normal place to go to at a time of upset at home, it can also be seen as a safe place for a teacher to use opportunities to teach about loss and death when the opportunity arises. The example given earlier of a class having the death of their gerbil explained is a good example of this. In the survey mentioned earlier, many junior school children said they felt death should be discussed with them as part of the school curriculum.

Some teachers can and do include death and bereavement in PSHE (Personal, Social, and Health Education) or RE (Religious Education). But the emotional processes of grief and dealing with our own grief requires more than simply knowing about rites of passage. The less it is taught in school, the greater will be the cost to health services and other publicly funded or voluntary resources for 'sticking plaster' remedial work.

Local bereavement organisations will often assist if approached, not only with providing support to a bereaved child (with parental permission) but in advising a school as to how to respond both with individual children, and with the whole school community if, for example a child or member of staff dies.

A survey in American High Schools on the benefits of 35 years of delivering such education (where the students had the option of taking this course) showed that the students who had elected this programme had supplementary benefits:

- Fear of change and loss were reduced
- The children involved performed better in other subjects than expected

- Communication within families improved.[22]

While it is useful to have a staff member trained in working with bereaved child the actions of the class teacher have the most immediate impact on a child on returning to school. Although one child may have been mistaken in assuming that his teacher would not have approved of him leaving the class when he needed to the fact that he did not believe her indicated a lack of trust, and may have come about because of the way the teacher expressed this permission.

A number of teachers told of being obstructed in helping children by overprotective parents. One of them reacted to the resistance of some parents to allowing their children to attend parental funerals, by setting up a bereavement support group that seemed to help the children by reassuring them that they were not unique either in losing a parent or in their grief. A Head teacher who had a 'dinner lady' with two children at the school die suddenly, was told by her husband that he did not want this talked about or any special mention of it. The Head decided that the interests of the whole school came first and held a special memorial service for her, which the father did not attend.

Teachers and other professionals often comment they are not trained in dealing with child bereavement, and so feel apprehensive of talking to children on this subject, so several organisations have produced educational material for children, teachers, parents, and friends on what to expect, and run training programmes for them. (See the list at the end) But unless proper death and bereavement education is introduced these can only address the issue on a fragmentary basis, and the hurt and loss of self-esteem and security will go on. New Zealand already has such a programme, while Greece is being funded by the EU to experiment with material developed in Baltimore (USA).

'I didn't go back to school the next day (after mother died), then on Thursday, the day after, I went back. I wanted to see my friends again, talk to my teachers and my friends. Everybody was really nice' (Ruth)

Chapter 7. Back to school – other children's reactions

The reactions of peer friends or relatives seemed to fall into three main categories; those which were helpful and supportive, those which were intended to hurt, and the third, comments or actions which were not intended to be hurtful but which proved irritating and at times rejecting.

The more positive experiences included Hazel's who was also motivated to return to school as soon as possible by the prospect of seeing friends.

> 'Madeleine (best friend) said "Sorry" and things like that' and continued 'My friend Jean, her mum and my mum were best friends, and she said "I miss my auntie" 'cos she were like her auntie'

Like others, Hazel also commented on the difference between her friends and her 'best friend' to whom she could say almost anything.

> 'My best friend I can talk to, but not just, like, friends'

Ruth made a similar point and said how it helped when her best friend said

> 'Just remember how much she (mum) loved you and how much you loved her'

Several children told of instances in which classmates or others had said some quite spiteful things. Pat for example;

> 'There's this girl in class. She called me…. (inaudible)…and she's very, very, horrible to me and she started saying, like, "You can't play 'cos you're not allowed, and everyone's got a mum and you haven't". So I said "It's not my fault Kath"'.

Jennie did not experience this against herself, but her best friend's dad died a few months after her own, and came across to her one day in the playground.

> 'I don't know what they said but she came over and told me they'd been picking on her about her dad. After they'd picked on her I told them to go away and stop picking on her, then we went and told our teacher who was on duty'

David too told of being picked on and insults;

> 'At school, it gets.... I run outside. Just a few days ago, this kid swore at me in the dinner queue. In olden days the boy meant "You haven't got a dad"'

Mac's story was told in the section on school issues, but it was clear that he felt particularly betrayed as the snide comments on the coach trip had come from someone he had seen as a friend. Jill sensed she was being got at by a group;

> 'They kept on calling me an orphan, even though they know my mother is still alive. They kept on repeating "Your dad's died, your dad's died". I don't know how they know'

Some reactions by other children were not intentionally hurtful, but caused embarrassment or a sense of being different, apart from others. Typical comment was by Jenny, who complained that people would keep looking at her as though she was different;

> 'If the teacher says something like, "Ask your mum to sign this form for the school trip" some people always turn around to look at me'

As if they expect you to burst into tears or fall ill? *Yes*

Pat recalled her irritations on the same theme, the irony being her friends thought they were being kind;

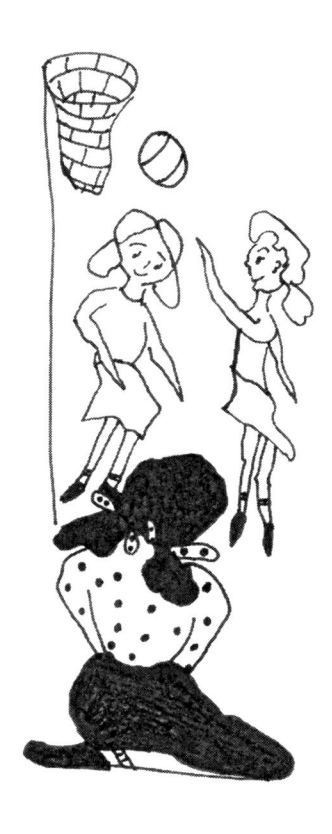

'When I went back to school, I thought it was going to be good, and everyone would just come up to me and say "How have you been?", and then let me play football or something, but I got about ten minutes and then they just started. They were patting me and saying "Do you want to sit down?"

Who the other children?

'Yes, I understand they wanted to help but I don't like being treated like I'm ......

Like you're sick or some thing?

yea, I didn't like it. It happened for about two months after that and I got really low, so I went and told. But they didn't know...... but even after that they were very sensitive with me and I didn't really like it although our teacher told them....... she doesn't want to be treated like a star!'

This last comment was similar to David's

'I just wanted to be treated as normal, like'

Although most wanted to get back to school and their friends, one or two stayed away longer

'I didn't want to come back because I were a bit

> upset on them days. I didn't want like crying then people asking 'What's up?' then I didn't want to tell them all the time' (Jill)

Five in total said they had experienced similar treatment, and one complained of teasing. Others were felt to be sympathetic but did not say much, as though they did not know what to say

> 'They weren't unkind, just didn't want to talk about dad. I think they thought it might hurt me'

Only Jimmy was away from school for an extended period, two months. The shock of his father's sudden death, he found, disabled him from concentrating on academic work. He was assisted to return eventually by being given small homework tasks, which at first he could not cope with but with which he slowly came to terms.

Conclusions and Recommendations

It is clear that some of the reactions of other children reflect fear that a similar disaster could happen to them, so they treat the bereaved child as if the tragedy is infectious. This comes across also in those situations where the others thought hey were being kind but proved annoying. Acting in this way frequently reflects the same experiences as bereaved adults who find that their friends have no language for grief.

The fear of being seen as different also raise a fear of being without friendships, the experiences of which psychologists tell us play a critical part in a child's acquisition of social identity and self esteem.

Comments from the girls highlight the only gender difference noticed in the research project. Girls laid a lot of emphasis on returning to school to be with their 'best friend'. Boys seemed more concerned with not appearing to be different by staying away. Even Mac's betrayal by his friend was related more as a cause of his anger in a specific situation and did not seem to influence how quickly he returned to school. His anger probably reflected the degree of emotional investment given to this friend.

What comes across is that the reactions of peers is as important for these children as those of family or teachers, while those of close or 'best' friends are vitally important to the child's sense of worth. The distinction between 'friend' and 'best friend' is emphasised, plus the use words of extreme emotion like 'hate' and 'like' to emphasise important differentials within the range of social contact. It is important not to downplay the importance of loss of friends or try to imply they are like standard replaceable parts by trying to comfort a child with such comments as 'Don't worry, you'll soon find another'.

I have often heard this tactic used when a child is faced with losing friends when moving house. It is more helpful to agree that the child will miss their friend and suggest they find a way to keep in touch. If practical, offer to have any special friend to stay over occasionally. Usually, as the child adjusts to their new environment their old friendships fade but at the time the break can be dramatic and create insecurity, especially when their new school community seems to have established friendships hard to break into. Losses are a normal part of growing up, and it is well to remember that the way we are taught to deal with them as children affects how we deal with them as adults.

Summary

When a child returns to school:
- Ensure that the head and class teacher are aware of what has happened.
- Teachers need to know how to recognise symptoms of extreme grief and behaviour caused by grief anger.
- Staff need to be alert for any sign of unpleasant speech or bullying.

- Ensure that a bereaved child is not treated in such a way as to feel they are singled out as 'different' from their peers.
- Ensure there is someone the child can talk to if needed.
- Be aware of the child's possible need to have short periods away from everybody.
- Asking a child as to the progress of a parent known to be very ill is appreciated and remembered.
- Do not assume that children will forget their hurt if it is not mentioned, or treat them as though nothing has happened.
- Locate helpful local and national resources – libraries, bereavement support organisations who usually have helpful literature for schools and many of whom will tailor short training programmes to suit school staff at minimal cost.

Chapter 8. Family influences

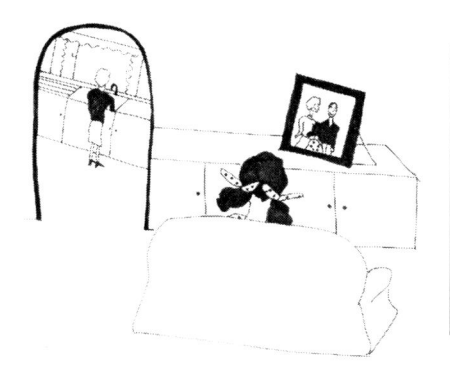

> 'If I talk to my dad it really upsets him' (Hazel)
>
> ' I don't talk to mum. She doesn't like it' (Mac)
>
> 'My dad never brings up the subject' (Sarah)

As can be seen from the illustration below, a child is at the centre of a system in which s/he is interacting with family, peers and others. So the death of one or more members influences the lives of them all, and also means that all the family will experience a shift in their relationships with each other and their sense of security.

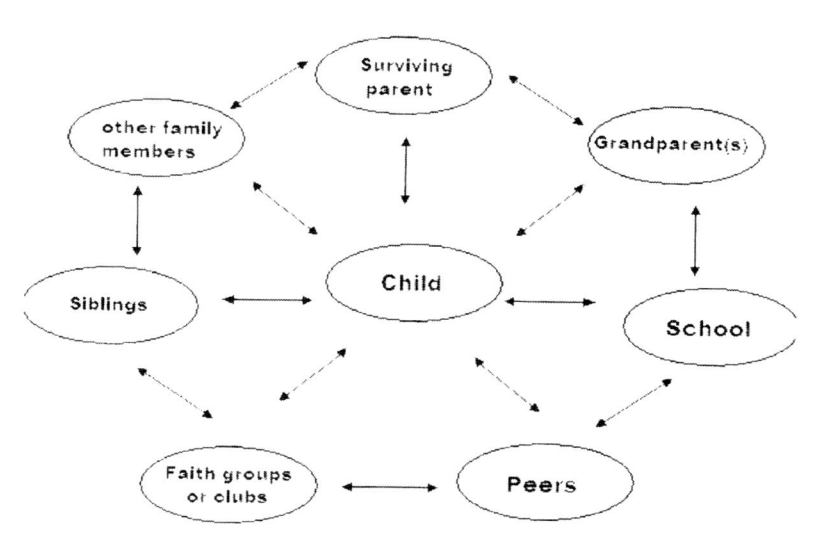

As such grief is a family event and not just for the individual child it raises all sorts of issues within the family such as communication, memories, fears and tensions between members plus happier experiences. When the death is of a key member i.e. a parent, all aspects of family life are affected.

Communication

Twelve of the children with a surviving parent felt able to discuss the deceased parent with the survivor. There were clear differences between families in the willingness to talk with children about their losses. Some typical comments on the reluctance of surviving parents to talk are given above. Others spoke of grandparents being similarly reluctant to talk.

> 'My dad and my gran don't talk, only Mrs S. (teacher). My gran doesn't like speaking about it' (Kevin)

Jill had a more positive experience:

> 'When my dad first died me and my mum and my sister used to talk about what it would be like without him'

Though she could not remember the content she thought it important and helpful.

Several children mentioned that it was easier to talk to their siblings than the surviving parent. Others told of being able to share grief

> 'We have our ups and downs, and we still cry together. It will be hard next month because the first anniversary is coming up. One of the hardest things is seeing all the photos' (Pat)

Memories

Alan had a very clear appreciation of his aunt and uncle (now his guardians) telling of their memories of his mother. David's mother died when he was just two years old. One of the things he valued from his dad, recently deceased, was that he and his older sister would tell him about his mum.

> *'In some ways I remember my mum. My dad and my sister used to tell me stories about her. When she died I was asleep. My dad went into the kitchen and closed the door. He started smashing plates.'*

Jill too spoke of missing her dad's stories

> *'My dad used to tell me about himself and my nanan, and he told me stories about when I was a little baby'*

> Are these memories important?

> *Oh yes. One was about when he was ten.'*

Fears and Tensions

Ronnie blamed his father for putting his mother under a lot of stress, and was convinced this had brought about her early death.

> *'He started going out. He was seeing someone else'*

Ronnie no longer sees his father and has no wish to. He was also happy not to be seeing his eldest brother and sister-in-law who took in him and another, elder brother when his mother died.

> *'They had a boy – Jimmy. We slept in a room with him. He started having really bad dreams like someone was chasing him, and they thought it was me'*

So he and his brother were put into care.

Sally was similarly angry with her father, who had left her when her mum was ill and had to go into hospital, so that the three children had to go into care. He does not seem to have made much effort to see the children, but when her mum died he came to see her the following weekend and brought his girl friend with him, to advise Sally that they had become engaged! Sally admitted that she'd had hopes of going back to their home all together and this really upset her. (This is similar to the situation of Mac referred to earlier in that the death of one parent removes all hope the child might have had of a family reconciliation).

The family fostering Sally and her brother were angry that the Social Workers placing them had no literature to help bereaved children and could give no help as to where to obtain any.

The potential for family reunions to provoke conflict was shown in Jill's experience.

> *'My uncle said "Are you happy?" but after that what made me upset was me mum and me uncle weren't friends any more and they aren't friends now'*

> They fell out did they, had a row? 'Yea, me dad's brother'

The effect of a family break up before the death of one parent had already affected three children. Mac, as I showed earlier was convinced that his dad would not have died if he had been at home. Sarah's parents had split up and she stayed with her mother but their home had been sold and she was already finding life more restricted by having to live with grandparents and share a room. Mother's death meant a move to another set of grandparents. She also admitted to other worries:

> *'It's strange not having her around all the time. I feel frightened at times – not having her. My fear now is that my dad will die. That would be really bad'*

Alan, by contrast, had lost his father at an early age, then his mother when he was 10. However, because his mother's sister and her family lived opposite them, but in a smaller house, he and his older sisters saw them all as part of their family so his aunt and her family moved across into his house.

> 'They moved here because this one's bigger, and we've got a bigger back garden'

David admitted anger with his parents who had both died:

> 'In some ways I feel angry with my dad and my mum for leaving us alone.... in some ways I feel guilty'

Jemma admitted missing being able to manipulate her dad.

> 'If my mum wouldn't buy me an ice cream I would always ask me dad'

> And you would usually get it? *(laughs)* .'Yes!'

She was aware however that the family had less income and knew her mum has to be careful.

Changing Roles and Relationships

> 'It feels strange, just the three of us. I miss her cooking!' (Jill)
>
> 'Mum pushed the table to the wall so that when we eat there isn't a spare chair where dad used to sit' (Michael)

This change in the relationship between the surviving members of a family after a death is illustrated by these and similar comments. It is common in many families that children relate to each parent differently and find they can say things to one that they find harder to say to the other. The death of the one that they favour talking to can leave a gap that is hard for a child to fill

> 'Some of the things that I did that made my dad laugh, my mum would take very seriously and tell me off for' (Michael)

Those in this study whose surviving parent had gone into a new relationship since the death of their parent seemed quite ambivalent about this. Jill, who was not told about her dad's death until she and the others arrived at church for his funeral is a good example.

> 'I live with my mum, and I'm alright because she's got a new boyfriend now and I'm moving house somewhere near dad's grave so I can just go and see him on my own' (Jill)

As many readers will have experienced just the opposite reaction from children when they have entered a new relationship, this cannot be taken as an assumed reaction. It may be partly to do with the fact that as her father had died no reunion was possible, whereas, as noted earlier, children whose parents have parted often hold a secret hope of their reunion which is dashed by a new relationship, but many have also known children unable to come to terms with such a new partnership even after a death.

One girl whose mother died found it inexplicable that whereas her parents had never had a row, when her father began a new relationship a year after her mother's death, the girlfriend and her father argued vehemently.

> 'About a year after my mum died my dad got a girlfriend. I'd never seen my mum and dad argue but they (dad & girlfriend) split up. It was scary' (Pat)

Other more positive changes were also noted

> 'Dad's really doing well. I didn't think he'd cope as well as he does. He never used to cook, he's fantastic now! He never ironed or hung washing out or went shopping, but he does all that now!' (Hazel)

This reflected practicalities experienced by other children, for good and bad. While Sophie acknowledged that her dad could cook quite well

> 'My mum could cook better. She could make chocolate cake!'

But Denzil missed the facility of kicking a football around with his dad.

> 'I don't like playing by myself. It's really boring'

Alan expressed a clear dichotomy in his reactions, owning up to both advantages and disadvantages arising from his mother's death, but nevertheless quite clear that he would prefer the disadvantages

> 'There's a big difference at home now. When my mum was here it was more crowded, now there's more room, especially as my sister has moved out as well. But I still want my mum here'

Conclusions and recommendations

All the evidence points to the usefulness to the child of the ability of the remaining parent being able to communicate with the bereaved child in a way that helps the child to adjust to their loss[23]. This is a major factor in limiting the amount of stress experienced by bereaved children at home or at school.

The fact that only 12 of the 23 with a surviving parent had been able to have such discussions, and that the others thought it more important to protect the surviving parent by not upsetting them by mentioning their dead mum or dad, means that these children are deprived in a way that will affect their adjustment. It also deprives them of the opportunities to receive anecdotes and memories about the deceased, memories which are held by the surviving parent and grandparents.

Jill related how much she appreciated the stories her dad told her about her grandmother, and herself as a toddler. David appreciated how his father and sister had told him stories about his mother who died when he was two, some of which would have been lost forever to him when his father died. The fact that the main thing Jennie remembered about her dad's funeral was the story of how her parents became engaged illustrates how important children find such stories. Openness, honesty, and inclusion in decision-making between a bereaved child and surviving parent (and grandparent) are positive contributors to a child's well-being.

No specific conclusions could be drawn from the children interviewed in the project as to whether an only child suffers more than a child with siblings. From the author's own experience of a competitive family much will depend upon the norms within a family with regard to the ability or practice among family members of giving each other support.

Asked to assist a family in which a boy of 8 years repeatedly bit his elder sister (following the death of their grandmother), the author had the boy colour a body outline to show where he felt different emotions. The lad coloured all his mouth and chin area bright red to indicate where he experienced anger. Asked whether this was why he bit his sister he said she repeatedly said that he did not love his gran as much as she did.

On her return from school the sister was challenged with the words

> *'I think we all know why he bit you don't we?'* She nodded.
>
> *'So you won't say that again will you?'* She shook her head
>
> *'I don't think we need to tell your mum and dad do we?'* Vigorous head shaking! She appreciated that her brother had not told tales on her to the parents.

Bereaved children are encouraged these days to open memory boxes with artefacts of the deceased, including photographs. This and similar activities come under the heading known now as 'Continuing Bonds', which acknowledges that trying to make an abrupt severance from someone loved makes little sense, and puts the emphasis on change and adaptation of the relationship with the deceased. This helps a child (or anyone else) to carry on while greatly saddened by the death of a loved while at the same time maintaining a sense of their continuing influence in everyday life. (25)

While obviously helpful, they can only contain the child's own memories, not those of previous generations, and it was unfortunate to hear that one or two could not talk to grandparents. Denying this service for a child shows more of a concern for one's own feelings and ability to cope than the child's needs. The danger also is that when a child does not say much because it does not want to see the parent or grandparent upset, the adult thinks the child does not care or is not interested and therefore not grieving. What is often needed is the opportunity to talk, if necessary starting away from the parent.

Conflicts and tensions are found frequently in bereaved families, so Jill's experience (her mother falling out with the brother of Jill's deceased dad) is not uncommon. It is clear Jill was saddened at this rift, which has broken their family link. I have known similar tensions at funerals and wakes, ranging from adult siblings elbowing each other aside at a crematorium in order to establish seniority in the seating, to hurling sausage rolls and pork pies along with abuse at a wake tea in a church hall.

Other tensions were caused by sheer lack of attention to practicalities on the part of those deceased who knew the children would be left parentless. When Ronnie's mother died, his elder brother and his wife took him and another brother into their home, only to put them out to fostering on the grounds that their own son was having nightmares. Similarly, David's father, although he had arranged fostering verbally with a neighbour of the same ethnic group, had left no evidence of this to satisfy Social Services, so David and his sister were subjected to three foster homes in a few months, (including some very unhappy experiences) while Social Services checked out the neighbour. Social Services cannot be blamed for needing to check out the neighbour and not just acting on hearsay. These experiences might have been avoided had the parents taken legal advice.

By contrast, Alan's mother had clearly made legal arrangements that enabled Alan and his sister to stay in their home and for her sister and her family to move in to continue an existing close relationship It is significant that Alan found he could talk freely to his aunt and uncle, and they shared their memories of his mother.

The fact is that children cannot be protected from the pain of loss, but if we do not deal with it with them we are not preparing them to deal with one of life's realities that they are going to come up against many times, and if unable to work through their period of grieving may suffer lasting emotional damage.[26]

Children pick up family disputes and tensions very quickly, and also take on the likes and dislikes of their parents through lack of knowledge of the truth. In the same way they model their reactions to death and bereavement on those of their parents and repeat these with their own children unless taught otherwise.

A useful tool for a surviving parent or other carer to use after the death of someone close is suggesting that the family are about to start a difficult journey that will take some time. Such journeys, even as holidays, need careful planning and realising that those who take part feel safer when going with other people rather than going by themselves. If youngsters are starting out on such a journey they would have hopes and fears that they would express and which the adults with them could deal with. Others have used the metaphor of a puppy being separated from its mother and litter for the first time, and being seen to be lonely and frightened in its new home.

Summary

Children who have one parent die while the other survives need:

- To be able to discuss the deceased with the surviving parent and have such artefacts and memory tokens as will enable the child to have an appropriate continuing emotional bond with the deceased
- To have the services of someone outside the family to talk to if needed
- To have the GP informed of the death, especially if the deceased was no longer with the family, and of any health matters that might arise from it.

If the child has no surviving parents:

- If in the care of Social Services and foster parents, having staff and carers who understand the needs of bereaved children or at least where to obtain information on these needs
- Ensuring that whoever is responsible for disposal of the belongings of the last parent consults the child over the distribution or disposal of photographs or other personal items that will enable a continuing memory or bond with the deceased.

Helpful Publications

There are some excellent books for children of all ages which have stories that help children understand both the concept of death and what they might feel and experience before and after the death of someone close. Such books are seldom found in ordinary bookshops. The organisations listed at the end of this book with their websites, hold such stories and will advise the most suitable if approached.

Chapter 9. Personal and Spiritual issues

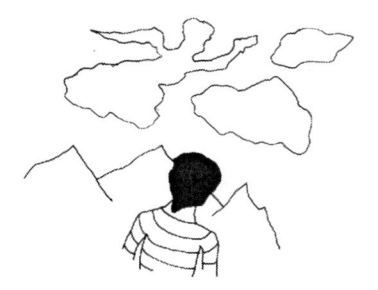

> *My gran said 'he's up there' (pointing upwards) (Mac)*
>
> *'My dad says they've gone up there' (Hazel)*
>
> *'He's in heaven' (Lucy)*

When reading the word 'spiritual' many people assume that what follows will be about religion. But the Concise Oxford Dictionary defines spiritual as *'relating to or affecting the human spirit as opposed to material or physical things'* whereas religion is something practised either in rites or/and in a way of life. Not everyone wants to be thought of as religious but there can be very few people without that human spirit which gives meaning and purpose, and also creates values. So while religion necessarily has a spiritual dimension, spirituality does not necessarily include religious practice.

Where are they now?

Views on life after death varied between one or two with fairly orthodox Christian beliefs, to a heaven defined as a place where the deceased participate permanently in the favourite activity they had in this life. For example Ruth

> *'My dad said she's probably gone shopping in a really posh shop, because she loved shopping'*

Jill told a similar tale:

> *'My auntie makes me laugh, because she says, now me nanan's died, her mum and me dad, all three of them have gone to the pub and got drunk.'(Jill)*

There was no indication that these children actually believed these suggestions, more the indication that the adults concerned did not know what to say when asked.

Melanie however was given a metaphor by her grandmother, with a distinctly Christian origin and which she clearly found helpful

> *'He's in Heaven. Because my grandma said, it's just his overcoat that's passed.*

But another adult had also clearly passed on an idea to her of her father's divine influence, which had a less orthodox message

> *'Daddy sent a dog down, because he died on 26th and the dog was born on 27th'*

Pat was more reflective, especially on the integrity of adults.

> *'Some people think she's gone and gone forever, but others think she's still with us. I don't know. Adults, they try to make you feel comfy, they say different things and you find out they are not true.'*

Julie reflected a view learned from her aunt that clergy often find in adults from ministerial practice, the idea that the deceased are 'up there watching us'

> *'I talked with my auntie on this. I think they are all together in heaven watching how good we are'*

'Oh, so they're keeping an eye on us?

'That's what my auntie tells me'

Does that make you 'gooder'?

> *'Well, it makes me a lot happier when you know they are sitting there. I just wish I was with them, but I don't want to go to heaven yet!'*

Are they still around?

Sixteen of the children felt the deceased was 'still around', especially in certain situations. Alan's comment was standard:

> 'I feel she's still around especially when we go out'

Pat, again, was more reflective: After her mother's funeral, which was entirely secular, she was aware of seeing her mother's face in a vision from her bedroom window the same night.

> 'People say they don't know whether she is with us. I still love her and it's a bit scary, but I know she wouldn't harm me. I just think sometimes - she's with us'.

Others sensed the presence of the deceased but felt that the idea was 'weird'. As Marilyn put it:

> 'I know he's not the same person or something or that I'd see him in the flesh sort of thing, I feel like he's alive, but he's not, it's pretty weird.'

Do you sometimes see faces of him? '*Yea*'

Do you worry about it sometimes?

> 'Sometimes it does scare me but I go to sleep anyway. Susie (counsellor) told me to say 'Would you stop doing this because it scares me'

Melanie spoke of 'dreams that are not really dreams'

> 'When I see him I run up to him and he's not there. I can see him but I can't touch him. It's upsetting but I'm all right'

Mabel reported similar experiences but did not feel scared:

> 'because I know he's my dad and he wouldn't hurt me'

Louise reported hearing noises upstairs when she knew there was nobody there, and felt it was her father's way of conveying 'I'm here'. But then she remembered:

> *'One of my uncles had died in the same year. He didn't like me much. I was frightened it might be him'*

Several children spoke of talking to the deceased:

> *'I tell her I love her with all my heart, and all that stuff' (Pat)*

> *'I talk to her sometimes in my room and tell her about school. I find that a comfort' (Hazel)*

> *I feel she's still near me. My friends say she is (Alan)*

David gave a unique view. He and his older sister had concluded that their parents had left them for a purpose:

> *'We think they knew they could not give us everything we needed and wanted to…..make sure we had advantages as we grew up, so we would be better off if they left us.'*

Conclusions and recommendations

Many of the beliefs and values stated would, from the perspectives of orthodox faiths, be classed as 'folk religion' i.e. beliefs based on popular myths, opinions, or perhaps superstitions, rather than creeds. Some such ideas can do more harm than good, for example the often quoted opinion 'God always takes the best ones first' mentioned previously. There is a clear sense with many of these youngsters that they derive some comfort from a belief in a deity and an afterlife.

The views expressed quoted above by David and his sister on the purpose of the deaths of both parents reflected thinking more in keeping with a teenager than an 11 year old, and they both expressed determination to make sure that this purpose was fulfilled by having worthwhile career ambitions.

Tensions can arise within families when a child professes a belief that is not shared by the parents, but in verbalising their disbelief to such children parents can cause additional distress by trying to remove a source of comfort that the child has found helpful. Ironically such parents are often among those who have refused to have their child christened or named as infants in any religious ceremony on the grounds that 'they can make up their own minds when they are older'.

The sense of the 'presence' of the deceased, frequently expressed by the children, of the person to whom they have been closely attached, is just as common among adults, as is the experience of believing they have 'seen' the deceased. It was also clear that while they were not happy about this experience, neither were they frightened.

A girl in her early 'teens, not part of the survey, kept seeing her deceased father carrying out his routines of winding all his clocks (of which he had several) in the house every day when she returned from school, and in her room at night. She was advised to try telling him, *'Look daddy, I shall always love you, but there is a place where you should be now, and it's not here. I am still here and your visits are upsetting me. Please go to wherever you are supposed to be'*

Ten days later asked how it went. *'Brilliant'*, she said, *I've only seen him once.'* asked 'What did you say to him?' she replied 'I said, *Dad, booger off. He's not been back since!'*

However, the same things do not help every child. One teenager, so desperate to establish contact again with her much loved daddy, consulted a spiritualist, again, not unknown among adults, but not advisable for children, specially if not accompanied by an adult of the same faith.

Summary

- If a child expresses a belief or faith give it the same rights to that belief that an adult would have. If it is clearly absurd, ask where they found it and what evidence there is for it.
- If they have an awareness of a 'presence' try not to dismiss this or use derogatory language ('rubbish, stupid, ridiculous').
- Ask the child if their experience frightens them, or if they think the presence will harm them. Point out that if they loved the person and they know the deceased loved them. the presence is not likely to harm them now
- Try to get trained help that knows how to deal with such experiences.
- If the family share a common faith, the use of prayer will help.
- There are a number of publications by organisations listed at the end that can be useful. Among them is the modern non-religious parable – story 'Water bugs and dragon flies'[26]
- Whether or not the family share a faith, a statement such as 'Your mum/dad will always be with us in one sense because our love for her/him and hers/his for us will always be with us' helps the child by expressing a truth. As one child in the Childhood Bereavement Network video interviews says

'You'll always remember them, even when you're old'

Chapter 10. Personal change and development

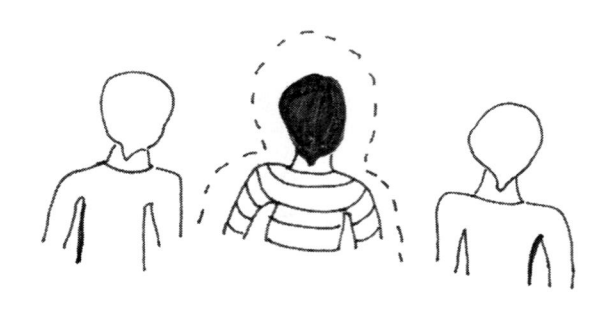

> 'The experience has changed me. I didn't think I would cope. I'm more confident now she's dead, and I wasn't confident before'   (Louise)

Several children reflected on their changed attitudes. Louise (above) saw changes in herself as very positive, with a clear indication of reduced dependency. Some saw a big change in their appreciation of the deceased:

> 'It changed how much I love her, because I used to love her a lot, but I love her even more now' (Pat)

> 'It makes you realise how close you are to someone, how much you loved them' (Ruth)

Jemma recognised that her behaviour had changed:

> 'I used to be more naughty when my dad was around, now I'm good'

Can you tell me why?

> When I'm naughty now, she like, gets upset'

She can't say 'Dad, deal with your daughter?'

(laughs) – No!'

Four children expressed the view that their self-esteem had been raised by their experiences, others implied it.

> Pat *'my dad says you've done well to get through all this'*
>
> So you feel proud of yourself?
>
> *Sometimes, yes, sometimes, no'*

David, who had lost both parents, been called names and bullied, and had been through some rough experiences in care, was self-affirming in a very unboastful way:

> *'Social Services classified my sister and me as young carers. I feel quite proud to say I was 9 – 10 years old and I've come through that much. I'm a reading tutor, I support charities, I do odd jobs.'*

Melanie reflected on her change of status as influencing her sense of being 'different'

> *'I feel different – they've got a daddy and I haven't. I have a person in my family who's died and there's no way anybody can change that.'*

Awareness of their reactions to the death being better than they had anticipated for themselves also came across.

> *I didn't think I would cope but even at school I feel included*
>
> *'I didn't think I would do so well especially in maths.' (Alan)*

Sarah noted that her increased confidence (arising from the affirmation given to her by an outside helper), enabled her to deal with conflict more easily and without fear.

> *'We played card games and did other exercises, so now, if someone says something nasty to me I will*

> say 'Please stop saying that'. Before I wouldn't say anything'

Sarah also felt confident in criticising the way adults deal with children following a death

> 'It's not helpful when they don't ask the children, like when a parent dies they just ask the grownups about everything and they make decisions without knowing.'

Conclusions and recommendations

Most children expressed a real anxiety about being seen as 'different' by others. But there was also a sense of knowing they *were* different and would have to live with this, at the same time recognising that the experience had also made them realise they were stronger and more self reliant than they had anticipated. When asked 'Looking back, if anyone had said beforehand that you would cope this well if your mum/dad died, would you have believed them?' without exception they said 'No'.

Adults often call this resilience, but there is also a view that these reactions are more than this. Resilience really means bouncing back to where you were beforehand, whereas most of these children expressed the view that their experiences made them feel older than their peers and more mature.[27] It was clear from their views of themselves that they felt they had grown up in dealing with something from which it is not possible to shield them and also that they resented any actions that prevented them dealing with their bereavement in a way that excluded them from showing their affection and respect for someone they loved.

The comments by Jemma quoted earlier of her awareness that her father's death meant a loss of family income showed a mature appreciation of her mother's message that although the family would not suffer great poverty, they would have to be careful with their finances.

Summary

- Children bereaved of a parent feel different to their peers but do not wish to be singled out as different.
- Actions such as the symbolism of lighting a candle on the birthday of the deceased or at Christmas with the actual expression of how much the person is still loved and remembered can help a child overcome feelings that their appreciation of the deceased was not appreciated sufficiently while they were still with them
- Many are aware of having come through a crisis better than they ever imagined they could have done, and being the stronger and more self reliant as a result.
- The adult (whether parent, teacher, social worker, or other) who is explicit in affirming and commending a child who comes through in this way helps the child's sense of worth and self esteem
- Children often see themselves as underestimated by adults.

Chapter 11 Help from outside the family

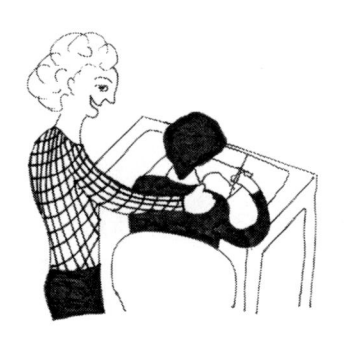

> 'Sometimes it's easier to talk to people outside. Sometimes, when you talk in the family, it makes you feel uncomfortable. So other people who aren't that close to you as your family, then sometimes, you feel more comfortable' (Ruth)

Eleven children in total had received help from four bereavement support organisations, while four others were clearly helped by school mentors who had been on training conferences or courses on child grief. As Pat put it

> *'It's easier to talk to somebody from outside'*

Ruth was more reflective;

> *'It does help to talk to people about things and not just be unhappy because when you don't talk to someone about problems then you feel yourself getting really depressed and just end up getting really lonely. So it's better to talk about problems you have.'*

Eric brought up an interesting and perceptive observation on this subject.

> *'they can't distract you so easily'*

In other words they won't change the subject.

Typical comments made to the author later, after the interviews, when asked how they had felt about talking to a stranger about the loss of their parent reflected in some cases the way many children are protective of their surviving parent.

> *'I knew that you wouldn't be upset talking about my mum'*

But not everyone wants to listen, as Sarah discovered:

> *'Many think it's like, frightening for me when I talk about my mum, but I'm like – it's not. Sometimes I talk to my teacher'*

Help from teachers or counsellors

Several children spoke with appreciation of time spent with teachers, feeling that their grief was being acknowledged sympathetically. One child, who had been shunted between relatives and schools in various parts of the country and finished up with foster parents, felt settled at the school where interviewed, and that the mentor had given him help and helped him to feel valued.

> *'Life has been better since I've had bereavement counselling' (Ronnie)*

Others talked about memory boxes, drawings, and scrap books they had made with the help of mentors, plus colouring exercises illustrating how their feelings had changed in the months since the death of their parent. Others showed dolls made of pipe cleaners, made by the mentors to provide comfort and receive whispered secrets at bedtime especially, when they found they were most prone to thoughts of sadness at their loss.

Even more important perhaps was the fact that three of them kept diaries that showed the changes in their emotions and other progress over several weeks. Of the eleven who had received help from support organisations only one had not seemed to benefit, apparently due to the anger still felt at his father's death, believing it to have been caused by his parents splitting up. Others were appreciative;

> 'I used to tell her about bullying and she helped me with that' (Pat)

Pat described other exercises to help her remember aspects of her mother's life and personality. I asked her how these helped her. She used a vivid metaphor.

> ''Well, you're kind of getting rid of your feelings and giving them to the person who died. All these little worries you have you just want to say to mum, that I'm keeping in a bottle, I just kind of undid the screw and it all came out, and it's quite nice actually'

An interesting view, and one which would hold for a lot of children, was given by Melanie. She was explicit as to how a support worker had enabled her to ventilate her feelings in a way she could not do with other people.

> 'Um, well, it's coming up to my daddy's anniversary, so we have done things together when it comes up to my daddy's anniversary'.

:I see, and that helps you does it?

> 'Yea. The way that she cares, and the way that she keeps stuff that I don't want anybody else to hear'

The value of art work, memory boxes, scrap books, games and exercises was mentioned by several children.

> 'I used to come up at night just to look at them (jar and memory box) and think about what me and my dad used to do and what kind of person he was' (Marilyn)

> 'I painted a picture of me and my mum in the park

> and that helped me get through that she wasn't here any more but I've still got memories of her' (Louise)

> 'The colouring and painting exercises helped me find out where I am with things like jealousy and anger. It's better than just talking' (Julie)

'The Grief Game' (Kingsley Publications) and similar non-competitive aids to reflection enable members of a family of all ages to sit down together to discuss different memories, plus thoughts and feelings in a way not otherwise likely to occur.

Weekend group residential meetings.

In addition to the above individual work, some children had attended meetings with other children to share experiences and carry out work together. Most appreciated this. Josh, for example who did not find much use for a chalk jar exercise but

> 'Sometimes we talked to each other about the person who died. It helped me move one step forward. So I didn't feel any different because everyone has had someone who died'.

Ricky too was explicit

> 'Well, quite recently we started coming here and meeting some other families who had lost their parents, or somebody really close, and that's been really good to find out what positions they've been in and then in the group we have some whose mum or parent had died say 3 – 4 years ago, and how they'd coped with things…..I think I would have found it harder if I hadn't gone.'

Mabel was more ambivalent about her experience as she found the start of the weekend difficult

> 'We did a candle ceremony. It was absolutely horrible, because everyone was crying, it was the worst experience ever'.

But she was pleased she persevered, and did not let this event prejudice her against the rest.

> 'Yea, it really did help me'

Despite all the crying ?

> 'Yea, because I was quite angry. I was quite angry that my daddy died, and I was still very angry at that camp, and one day I find out we were going to be make clay discs, and we weren't told what for, so I just made these little clay discs and made sad faces and glad faces and angry faces and stuff, and then we all had to have them in our hands when they were dry and we had made a lot more and kept them over obviously and we had about 4-5 discs in our hands that were dry and we walked out on to the field, and all we could see was this big wall,
>
> Next thing we knew we were told to chuck all these discs at the wall to let out anger out and we were just smashing everywhere, it was so funny.'It got all our anger out'

Conclusions

The school mentors mentioned and many of the volunteers from support organisations were not professional grief specialists. They were trained in the usual way and to the standards expected from voluntary organisations, which obviously would not include the same theoretical base as a more academic or professional course. Yet they evidently managed to achieve recognisable movement in the grief process for these children in the majority of cases and avoided the danger that many people who claim to feel better through talking to a counsellor have not actually moved.[28] They also assisted at very practical levels important to the children such as bullying.

Some of those who staff support organisations and who run the residential weekends are professionally trained and have qualifications from recognised institutions. It is difficult to draw any definite conclusions as to the differences more experienced or more professionally qualified counsellors might have made since the needs of the children are so variable. Those who research these matters did conclude that such interventions offered to children seem to be the only grief interventions that could be proved to be beneficial in terms of diminishing grief related symptoms.

What anybody involved with bereaved children does need to bear in mind is that nearly a quarter of all such children might need help for the first time two years after a death (29)

What is not helpful is, if a child is having 'flashbacks' i.e unhappy and unwanted memories intruding and upsetting, is telling them to think of something else less frightening or unhappy. The author heard a survivor of the Abervan disaster recount 30 years later how he had been given the advice a few weeks after the tragedy, when having flashbacks, to think of parties and games. Having already told the person saying this that all the children he might have played or had a party with were dead he was left wondering who needed help more, himself or the speaker.

It was clear from stories told that some children held a lot of anger, about such things as family break up before the death or as a result of the death. Unless this is dealt with remedial work may not be helpful.

Chapter 12 Overprotection

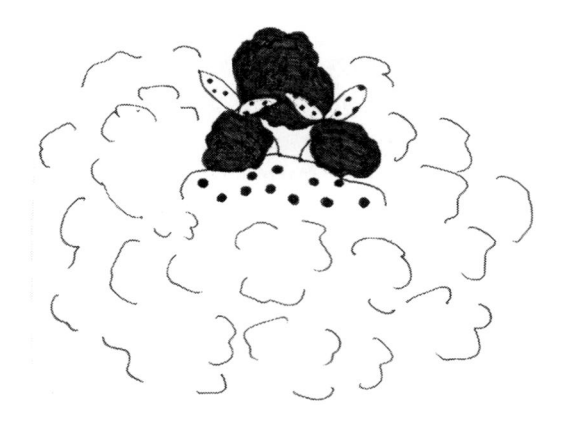

Just over 40 years ago a reputable study of childhood development (31) concluded

> 'People with high self esteem are so equipped because parental expectations represent a belief in their child's adequacy and a conviction that it has the ability to perform in whatever way is required to succeed.
>
> When set at reasonable levels, they represent a parental vote of confidence and provide a clear indicator that what is desired is attainable, thereby giving courage as well as direction. This confidence that one can deal with adversity, realise personal strivings, and gain respect and attention, is likely to be self-fulfilling by the persistence and poise it engenders, and by the demands it imposes on others.'

The study went on to point out that when a parent is overprotective and 'cocoons' a child, the child remains dependent and has poor self esteem.

When parents do allow their children to be exposed to a situation which is not abnormal or life threatening where they may cry, whether it be a funeral or a competition in which they may not succeed, they are allowing them to test their personal adequacy, and not live in an artificial environment in which they are protected and restricted. Tears are, after all, part of healing, not part of the hurt, and such children are likely to be more creative, with higher self-esteem and greater independence than those cocooned.

So while our first concern must always be for the protection of a child, to this must be added a concern for *over* protection. Parental acts of over nurturing can lead to a loss of abilities to regulate a life away from the nurturer, and bring about what is known as 'learned helplessness'.

When someone has low self esteem this can be seen in their low expectations for themselves, their belief hat they cannot succeed in anything they have not done before, and their anticipation that they will be rejected. When a parent has low expectations for their child these feelings are reinforced. So a child with low self esteem is unlikely to believe that his/her personal actions can have a favourable outcome, that she/he can effectively cope with adversity, or is worthy of love and attention, thus sapping courage or hope of dealing with problems that must inevitably be confronted.

This lack of parental confidence in children's ability to cope, was part of the experience of the author in parish work when trying to convince parents that a child should at least have the opportunity to decide for itself whether or not to attend the funeral of someone who has clearly been close to them. Frequently the response would be 'it's not fair to expect a child to cope with a funeral.'

When it is pointed out that many adults have lived for years in anger at being excluded, with feelings of guilt at not having said a proper 'goodbye' by being sent to school on the day of their mother or father's funeral, and that the opportunity to say 'goodbye' will not be there in the same way again, the reply is usually 'he'll understand when he's older'. The truth is – indeed he will understand and be even more annoyed.

It is not only parents that can underestimate a child's strength in adversity. In starting this study, the author was warned that children would feel safer with interviews in their homes rather than at school, and that junior schools do not have the facilities for such interviews, a view that seemed sensible enough.

In the event, of the children who were contacted through schools, 50% preferred to be interviewed at school rather than at home as they felt this would be less upsetting for the remaining parent. Those with foster parents were particularly strong in speaking of the school as a 'safe' place. The schools themselves went out of their way to make the facility available, in some cases teachers giving up their own rooms.

Members of the university ethics committee then expressed the view that if children were interviewed at school they could not be expected to return to class immediately afterwards. But in the same way as the interviews revealed that most children wanted to return to school as quickly as possible after the death of their parent so as to seem 'normal' to their friends and peers, and to have their company, none of those interviewed at school expressed any wish to opt out after the interview, though their teachers knew what was happening and kept a cautionary observance of them.

This demonstrates what one writer described as 'children's ability to put grief down and pick it up again'.

Summary

Children who had experienced disruption over several months recognised that school counselling had helped them become more stable.

- Several counselled at school could see the evidence of their progress from diaries, collages and drawings.
- Children counselled by other agencies could articulate the benefits they had received from the experience.
- The most important factor seems to be that any such support activities are age related.

It is clear from the data that there are some children who have a definite need to talk to somebody outside of their family or others close to them, and, as Melanie put it '*to hold those things that I don't want anybody else to know*'. This is not because of the incompetence of parents or others, but because, like the rest of us, there will be some matters connected with grief that the individual does not want to share with their nearest and dearest. The need for trained supporters who can listen and deal with such children is therefore vital if they are to progress through grief without storing up personal baggage that will eventually require professional help either medical or psychological.

Several authorities emphasise that the most important part of any grief support with a child is to help the child tell his or her story, and this will require suitable age related materials. The range of these in use in helping children indicates that the mentors and counsellors understand this. Children observe many things they cannot name (29), and one of the roles for support workers is to enable them to find the language to identify their own and others' reactions and thereby begin to understand them. It seemed highly significant to me that the two children who were among those best able to describe the ways in which the interventions of the support worker had helped them were in a school that has a teacher who specialises in emotional literacy.

The research and survey referred to throughout this book does seem to show a gap between the knowledge gained through research and experience coming from the bereavement specialists, and other sections of society. The quotations given also point to gaps in training in children's bereavement needs for social workers, teachers, and clergy.

There is also evidence that some of those involved in helping children seem unaware of children's needs to revisit their loss as they mature (32) This is also the case with teachers, social workers and others as shown by their reluctance to allow such children to be interviewed There was a general underestimation of children's strength and courage, as evidenced by the responses to requests for help from an NHS County Research Ethics Committee, and a number of counselling organisations, that asking children questions about bereavement would be harmful.

The author is therefore very grateful to those parents, teachers and organisations that did have such understanding and allowed access to talk to the children quoted here. But the author's most heartfelt thanks go to the truly wonderful youngsters who have been so frank and trusting in their responses to questions and about their fears, hopes and feelings. The response from almost every one of them to the question '*Would you like to say why you agreed to take part?*' was the same.

> '*If it will help other children to get through this, I will be pleased*'

The author has been amazed at the variety of experiences and practices recounted during this investigation, and left with the query and worry - if this is what has been uncovered by such a small sample, (found with difficulty, and random) what is happening to the rest of the 18,000 under 18's who lose a parent each year as well as nearly two million who have lost another attachment figure in the past 10 years? Every second person spoken to about this project seems to have their own story of exclusion or insensitivity, some related from experiences 50 years earlier.

Some writers speak of the 'anti-child bias' in our society (33), while others tell of studies in which physically handicapped children did not expect their views to be taken seriously (34). While the reactions of some adults are more to do with their own fears rather than being directly 'anti-child' the effect is to the detriment of the child, and as pointed out in the opening chapter for some children this has led to deep frustration and anger, with subsequent behavioural problems and school exclusion.

Chapter 13. General Conclusions

While there is increasing knowledge and appreciation of bereavement issues for children among voluntary and professional groups involved in their care, it is evident from the children interviewed that only a small number of families follow recommended practice, mostly through intuition or inherited parenting skills rather than education.

While the psychological processes and pain of grief are mostly unavoidable, it is also clear that the actions of the adults around bereaved children are a major contributory factor towards what is often referred to as a healthy progress through grief.

It is clear from the information gained from the author's study, as recounted in these notes that some children go through unnecessary additional pain or distress through ignorance of these factors by those who take decisions for these children, in many cases without consulting them. Ironically, many actions that make matters worse for a child, such as refusing the option to attend a funeral, are often taking thinking that this is in the best interest of the child.

On a positive note however, the encouraging factor that has shone through this whole project has been the way that so many children have coped with the problems caused by such things as lack of contingency planning by deceased parents when finding themselves orphans, school bullying and lack of sensitivity by teachers or carers, yet have come through stronger than when they started, and enhanced in self esteem by the way they have coped.

For the benefit of those who might want to embark on further studies into this subject, the sources from which some of the information was taken are numbered in the text and listed at the back of the book.

In addition, for those who might wish to pursue investigations further by interviewing children, there is an appendix available from the address on page iv showing:

- The ethical issues that have to be taken into account and which are required by university ethics committees, together with references as to where to find details of these.
- Some of the barriers that were put up by gatekeepers (Head teachers, social worker managers, counselling organisations, a County Medical Ethics Research committee) and how these were either overcome or proved an obstruction.
- Notes on how the interviews were structured and children's initial shyness or hesitancies were overcome.
- A further list of references relating to research issues.

This appendix can also be ordered from:

www.briancranwell.co.uk

Useful organisations for help with children and/or publications

Such publications include recommendations for parents, teachers, carers and grief support workers, where to find programmes for helping children or for training support workers, help cards, story or work books for children across the age ranges that can assist their understanding of grief.

Child Bereavement Charity. West Wycombe Buckinghamshire 01494 446648

www.childbereavement.org.uk

Childhood Bereavement Network. London. National Children's Bureau. 020 78436041

www.ncb.org.uk

Gone Forever Trust, Sheffield.

www.goneforever.org.uk

Winstons Wish, The Clara Burgess Centre, Cheltenham
www.winstonswish.org.uk

The author wishes gratefully to acknowledge the assistance of the following in locating parents and children to take part in this study. In doing so they have without exception followed the ethical and confidentiality protocols recommended for such research.

The charities listed above

The Laura Centre, Leicester

Cruse Bereavement Care Rotherham Branch

Derby Diocesan Education Office

Sheffield Diocesan Education Office

Leicester Diocesan Education Office

Beck Primary School Shiregreen, Sheffield

Ballifield Primary School Handsworth, Sheffield

Deepcar St John's C of E Primary School, Sheffield

Hunters Bar Junior School, Sheffield

Oughtibridge Primary School, Sheffield

Reignhead Junior School, Beighton, Sheffield

Woodhouse West Primary School, Sheffield

Gilmorton C of E Primary School, Leicester

Wigston All Saints C of E Primary School, Leicester

(Endnotes)

References

1. Cranwell B (2007) Bereaved children's perspectives on what helps and hinders their grieving. *Child Bereavement Charity, West Wycombe*

2. Meltzer H., Gatward R., & Ford T. (2000) *The mental health of children and adolescents in Great Britain* Social survey Division of the Office of National Statistics

3. Black, D., (1993) *Highlight no. 120: Children & bereavement.* National Children's Bureau

4. Rolls E & Payne S (2003) Childhood bereavement services:. A summary of UK provision *Palliative Medicine 17 pp 423-432*

5. Op Cit 2

6. Silverman, P.R., & Worden, J.W., (1992) Children's reactions in the early month after the death of a parent *American Journal of Orthopsychiatry 62, 93 –104*

7. Op Cit 2

8. Rutter M., (1966) *Children of sick parents* London. Oxford University Press

9. Sweeting H, West F, Richards M (1998) Teenage family life, lifestyles and life chances: associations with family structure, conflict with parents and joint family activity. *International Journal of Law, Policy and the Family;*12 (1); 15-46

10. Goldman L., (2000) *Life and Loss* Philadelphia. Accelerated Development Inc.

11. Dyregrov A. (1990) *Grief in children: A handbook for adults* Jessica Kingsley Publishers. London

12. McArthy, J.R., Jessop, J., (2005) *The Impact of bereavement and loss on young people.* Joseph Rowntree Foundation

13. Waskett, D.A. (1995) Chairing the child – A seat of bereavement In Smith, S.C. & Pennells M (Ed) *Interventions with bereaved*

	children.London. Bristol. Pennsylvania. Jessica Kingsley Publishers Ltd.
14	Herbert, M., (1996) *Supporting bereaved and dying children and their parents* Leicester. The British Psychological Society.
15	Faulkner, A (1994) *When the news is bad.* Stanley Thorne, Cheltenham, England
16	Parkes, C.M., & Weiss R.S., (1983) *Recovery from bereavement*, New York. Basic Books
17	Fristad, M.A., Cerel, J., Goldman, M., Weller, E.B. & Weller, R.A.(2001). *The role of ritual in children's Bereavement.* OMEGA Vol 42(4) 321 – 339, 2000 - 2001
18	Black D. (1993) The bereaved child: An overview. *Supporting Bereaved Children &Families.* Sargoni et al (Ed). Cruse Bereavement Care
19	Silverman, P.R., & Worden, J.W., (1992) Children's understanding of funeral ritual *Omega: Journal of Death and Dying*, 25, 319 – 331
20	Ibid
21	Lowton K., & Higginson J.H., (2003) Managing bereavement in the classroom: A conspiracy of silence? *Death Studies* , 27: 717 - 741
22	Stevenson, R.G. (2004) Where do we come from? Where do we go from here? Thirty years of death education in schools. *Illness, Crisis and Loss.* **12**(3); 231-238
23	Wormbrod, M.E.T., (1986) Counselling bereaved children: stages in the process. *Social Casework,* pp 351 – 358
24	Op Cit 14
25	Riches, G., & Dawson P (2000) *An intimate loneliness: Supporting bereaved parents and siblings.* Buckingham. Oxford University Press
26	Stiickney D., (1982) *Water bugs and dragon flies* London. New York. Continuum
27	Schuurman, D., (2002) The club no one wants to join. *Grief Matters. August 2002. The Centre for Grief Education. Australia.*
28	Griffin J.,& Tyrrell I., (2002) *Psychotherapy, counselling, and the human givens* Chalvington UK H G Publishing for European Therapy Studies Institute. Organising Ideas No 2,

29	Worden., J.W., & Silverman, P.R.,(1996). Parental death and the adjustment of school – age children. *Omega 33: 91 – 102*
30	Silverman, P.R., (2000) *Never too young to know: Death in children's lives* London. Oxford University Press
31	Coopersmith, J (1967) *The antecedents of self-esteem* W.H.Freeman & Co
32	Jewett, C.,(1994) *Helping children cope with separation and loss.* London. Free Association Books Ltd
33	Alderson, P., (1995) *Listening to children; Children, ethics and social research.* Barkingside. Barnados
34	Watson, N., Shakespeare, T., Cunningham-Burley, S., Barnes, C., Corker, M., Davis, J., &Priestley, M, (1999).*Life as a Disabled Child: a qualitative study of young people's experiences and perspectives.* Universities of Edinburgh & Leeds

About the Author

Brian Cranwell, a retired clergy member, was a bereavement support worker for 20 years, training and supervising others in the same work. For the last 15 years of this he worked with bereaved children and trained others for the same function.

Entering late into church ministry after a career that included industrial relations management, training and management development, and management consultancy, he was dismayed to find how frequently children were left out of information about the impending death of someone they loved (and consequent lack of opportunity to make their farewells) and excluded from gatherings of family and friends for the funeral.

On approaching retirement he discovered that although a great deal of useful information had been written on the subject by professionals, nobody had taken the direct views of children so set about and successfully completed a child centred research programme supervised by Sheffield Hallam University, for which he was awarded the Degree of MPhil.

This book is intended to make the results of that research accessible to anyone who has responsibility for bereaved children - parents, foster parents, social workers, teachers, and clergy. The book is therefore not written as an academic work, the main emphasis being on the experiences and stories of the children.